THE IMMUNE SYSTEM DIET AND RECOVERY PLAN

Ultimate Cookbook with Natural Recipes to Boost Your Immunity, Prevent Disease and Stay Healthy

Tiffany Shelton

Disclaimer

The recipes and information in this book are provided for educational purposes only. Please always consult a licensed professional before making changes to your lifestyle or diet. The author and publisher shall have neither liability nor responsibility to anyone with respect to any loss or damage caused or alleged to be caused directly or indirectly by the information contained in this book. All trademarks and brands within this book are for clarifying purposes only and are owned by the owners themselves, not affiliated with this document.

Images from shutterstock.com

CONTENT

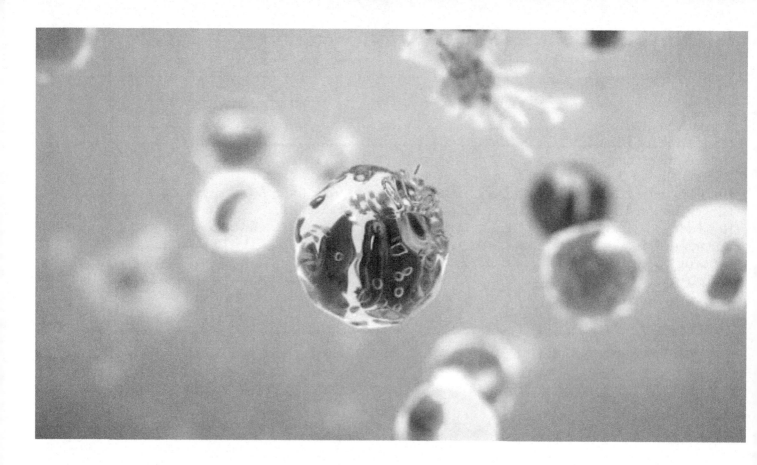

INTRODUCTION

Our immune system protects us from germs. Our body is constantly attacked by bacteria, viruses, fungi, and protozoa, and our only defense against them is our immune system. Therefore to protect ourselves is to support our immune system. And that's exactly what this book is about!

You will find out how the immune works and how you can make it stronger, how you can prevent diseases, discover what food is best or worst for your immune system and what vitamins and minerals are essential for its proper work.

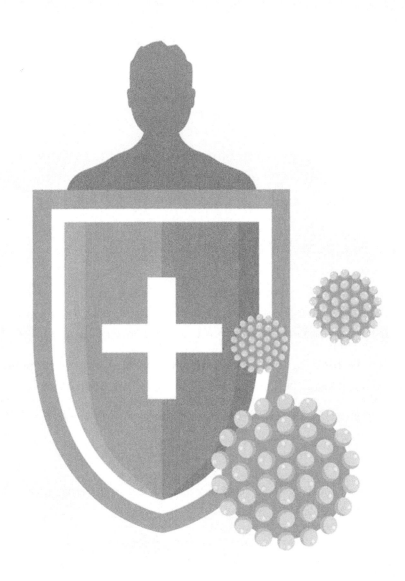

CHAPTER 1. ALL ABOUT YOUR IMMUNE SYSTEM

WHAT IS THE IMMUNE SYSTEM?

The immune system is a large network of cells, tissues, and organs that function together to protect our body from foreign body attacks. These invaders are microbes — microscopic, infection-causing organisms such as bacteria, viruses, parasites, and fungi. The human body provides an ideal environment for many microbes to survive, so of course they want to invade it. The immune system keeps them out, but when it doesn't work correctly or fails, the immune system starts to seek them out and destroy them.

The immune system is able to recognize and remember the countless intruders and produces cells and secretions that can defeat each of them so our body is safe again.

It works so effectively thanks to a dynamic communication network. In our body, there are millions of cells that move all around the body, passing information from one point to another. When they receive an alarm, the cells start to produce an effective weapon – it's strong and powerful chemicals. The cells can also regulate their behavior and growth that makes them very adaptive to different conditions.

We wouldn't be able to fight a huge variety of microorganisms or harmful changes inside the body without our immune system. Its main tasks are:

- fight and remove disease-causing pathogens such as bacteria, viruses, parasites or fungi.
- defeat disease-causing changes in the body.

As long as the immune system is running properly, you won't feel that it's there. But if it stops working smoothly because it can't fight some aggressive pathogens or it's weak, you will get sick.

HOW THE IMMUNE SYSTEM WORKS

The immune system is necessary for human survival. Without it, our body is fully open to attack from bacteria, viruses, parasites, and more. This massive network of cells and tissues is continually on the alert for threats, and if an intruder is detected, a dynamic assault is set up.

The immune system is distributed across the body and includes several kinds of cells, muscles, enzymes, and tissue. Damaged cells are also detected and destroyed by the immune system.

The immune system's work is expansive and consists of many parts.

White blood cells

Another name for white blood cells is leukocytes. These cells circulate in lymphatic tissue and blood vessels that parallel the arteries and veins.

Leukocytes are always on regular monitoring for pathogens. Once they reach a target, they begin to replicate and transmit signals to other cell types to do the same thing.

White blood cells are located in lymphoid organs. These include the thymus, spleen, bone marrow, and lymph nodes. There are two main types of leukocyte:

1. Phagocytes

These cells cover and consume toxins and break them down and destroy them efficiently. There are several types of phagocytes:

- neutrophils — the most common type that attack bacteria
- monocytes — the largest type that has several functions
- macrophages — monitor pathogens and remove dying and dead cells
- mast cells — protect from pathogens and help to heal wounds

2. Lymphocytes

Theses cells help the body identify former threats that have again entered the body. Lymphocytes are produced by the bone marrow. Part of them stays in the marrow to develop into B lymphocytes (alert T lymphocytes and produce antibodies), and another part goes to the thymus to transform in T lymphocytes (alert other leukocytes and destroys damaged cells in the body). These two types have different roles:

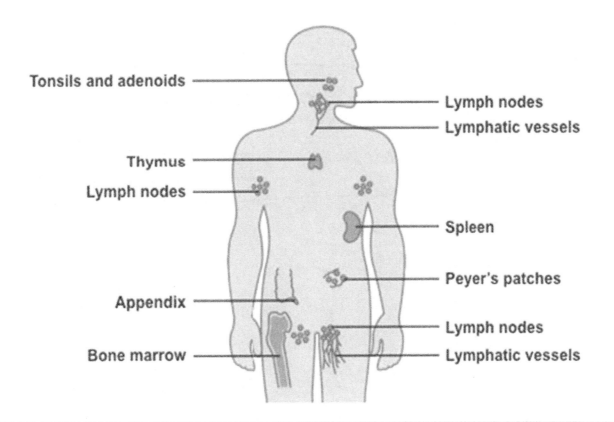

MAIN PARTS OF IMMUNE SYSTEM

The immune system organs are called **lymphoid organs** because they produce lymphocytes.

Bone marrow is the soft tissue at the deep core of the bones. It is the highly reproductive source of all blood cells, including white blood cells that become immune cells.

The thymus is located behind the breastbone; it is the place where T lymphocytes mature.

Blood vessels serve as one of the main routes for lymphocytes to travel throughout the body. Another route through the system is **lymphatic vessels** that parallel veins and arteries. Blood and lymphatic vessels are exchanged between cells and fluids, allowing the last one to control invading microbes in the body. Also, the lymphatic vessels carry a clear fluid, or lymph, that bathes tissues of the body.

Small **lymph nodes** are situated along the lymphatic vessels, with clusters in the armpits, abdomen, neck, and groin. Every lymph node is loaded with compartments where immune cells congregate and identify the antigens.

Peyer's patches are the structural units of gut-associated lymphoid tissue which are responsible for endocytosis and transport into intraepithelial spaces.

The **spleen** is located in the upper left of the abdomen. It contains specialized compartments where immune cells gather and work, and serves as a meeting ground when immune defenses face antigens.

Clumps of lymphoid tissue can be found in the airways and lungs, the linings of the digestive tract — territories that function as gateways to the body. These tissues include the **adenoids, tonsils, and appendix.**

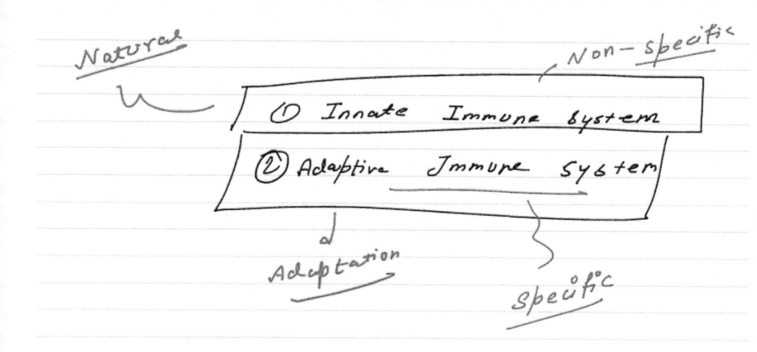

TYPES OF IMMUNE SYSTEM

Our immune system can be divided into two subsystems: **adaptive immunity** and **innate immunity.** Both these systems are closely connected and work together once a harmful substance or pathogen triggers an immune response.

The **adaptive immune system** produces antibodies and uses them to fight particular germs that our body has come into contact with before. This phenomenon is called an acquired or learned specific immune response. Thanks to the adaptive immune system that always learns and adapts, our body can fight viruses or bacteria that mutate over time.

You're born with **innate immunity** that consists of barriers in and on the body that protect from foreign threats. Skin, stomach acid, enzymes (found in tears, skin oil, and mucus) are the components of innate immunity. There are also a few elements of innate immunity found as chemical substances called interleukin-1 and interferon.

The innate immune system is a general defense against harmful substances and germs, so it's also known as the non-specific immune system. It basically fights using immune cells such as natural killer cells and phagocytes. The main task of this immune system is to fight injurious microbes and substances that enter the body through the digestive system or skin.

Immune Tolerance

Immune tolerance is the ability of B or T lymphocytes to ignore the body's own tissues. Scientists are trying to find out how the immune system knows when to ignore or respond.

Central tolerance occurs during lymphocyte development. In each immune cell's early life, it is exposed to a huge amount of self molecules in the body. If it hasn't fully matured and meets these molecules, the encounter starts an internal self-destruct process to kill the immune cell. It is called 26 clonal deletion that helps ensure that T cells and B cells do not mature and invade healthy tissues.

CHAPTER 2. DISEASES

The immune system's overactivity can take many forms, including autoimmune or allergic diseases. Underactivity of the immune system can make people vulnerable to infections that can be life-threatening in some cases.

AUTOIMMUNE DISEASES

Sometimes the immune system loses its identification ability, and the body starts to produce antibodies and T cells against its own cells and organs. Disoriented antibodies and T cells, as they are known, cause a huge variety of diseases. For example, T cells that attack pancreas cells cause diabetes, when at the same time, a rheumatoid factor (autoantibody) is common for people with rheumatoid arthritis.

Scientists can't say what exactly causes autoimmune diseases, but do not exclude the role of multiple factors such as sunlight, viruses, drugs – common parts of the environment that can damage normal body cells. Hormones may play a role too, and more for women than for men. Also, we cannot ignore heredity.

Diabetes

Diabetes mellitus is a metabolic disease that causes high blood sugar, also known as diabetes. One of our hormones, insulin, transfers sugar to cells from the blood to store or use it for energy. Your body can't properly use insulin effectively or produce enough to function correctly with diabetes.

If you don't treat high blood sugar, it can damage your kidneys, eyes, nerves, and other organs.

There are a few types of diabetes:

Type 1 diabetes	An autoimmune disease. The immune system destroys cells in the pancreas, where insulin is made. About 10% of diabetics have this type of disease.
Type 2 diabetes	The body becomes immune to insulin, so sugar builds up in the blood.
Prediabetes	The blood sugar is higher than it should be, but it's not enough for a diagnosis of type 2 diabetes.
Gestational diabetes	Blood sugar is high during pregnancy. This type of diabetes is caused by the placenta that produces insulin-blocking hormones.

Psoriasis

Psoriasis is a chronic autoimmune disease that provokes skin cells to build up rapidly. As a result, scales form on the surface of the skin. Common symptoms are redness and inflammation around the scales. Typical psoriatic scales ripen in thick, red patches and have a whitish-silver color. These patches also may crack and bleed.

Growing deep in the skin, the cells rise to the surface. After a while, they fall off. The skin cell's life cycle is one month. When you have psoriasis, the life cycle of skin cells is disrupted, and the production process is over after a few days. Skin cells cannot fall off because of a lack of time. This overproduction causes the buildup of skin cells. Skin scales usually appear on elbows, knees,scalp, hands, neck, feet, and face.

Less typical types of psoriasis appear on the mouth, the nails, and around genitals.

INFECTIOUS DISEASES

Infectious diseases are caused by micro-organisms — such as bacteria, viruses, or fungi. There are a lot of organisms that live on and in our bodies. They're harmless, and some of them are even helpful. Yet, in other conditions, some organisms can trigger the disease.

Signs, causes, and symptoms depend on micro-organisms that caused your disease. Though most common symptoms are fatigue and fever.

Direct contact

Infectious diseases easily spread because of their ability to be passed by direct or indirect contact. Examples of direct contact include:

- **Animal to person.** If you have been scratched or bitten by an infected pet or animal, you can contract a harmful and sometimes fatal infection. Be careful while handling your cat's litter box, as you may get a toxoplasmosis from animal waste.
- **Person to person.** This contact happens when a person with the virus or bacterium touches, sneezes, or coughs on someone who isn't infected. These microbes can also spread through sexual contact. The person who spreads the infection can have no symptoms and signs of the disease, but may simply be a carrier.
- **Mother to child.** A pregnant woman can infect her unborn baby with a virus or bacterium germs that lead to diseases. Some of them pass through breast milk or the placenta. Microbes in the vagina may be transmitted to the baby during birth too.

Indirect contact

A large number of germs lay on a doorknob, tabletop, or faucet handle. When you handle a doorknob touched by someone ill, you can pick up the microbes he or she left behind. Do not touch your mouth, nose, eyes before washing your hands, or you can get an infection.

Insect bites

Some infections can be passed by insects— fleas, mosquitoes, ticks, or lice. Mosquitoes can be carries of the West Nile virus or malaria. Deer ticks carry Lyme disease.

Food contamination

Disease-causing microbes may infect you through contaminated water and food. The transmission mechanism allows microbes to be spread to a lot of people through a single source. Escherichia coli, for example, is a bacterium that can be found in unpasteurized fruit juice or undercooked meat.

Bacterial Infections

Many different kinds of bacteria can make you ill. Bacteria can infect any part of the body, and can also spread throughout your blood, triggering the sepsis.

You may experience common symptoms, such as fatigue, chills, and fever when you have a bacterial infection. Also, you may feel other effects like example, swelling, pain, organ dysfunction, and redness.

Bacterial infections are triggered by the transmission of bacteria. You can be infected with bacteria from people, through the environment, drinking contaminated water, or eating contaminated food.

If you have a weak immune system or take immunosuppressive medication, you may be more susceptible to developing a serious bacterial infection — even from those types of bacteria that are normally innate to your body.

Bacterial infection	Type of infection	Description
Tuberculosis	Contagious disease	Caused by the Mycobacterium tuberculosis bacteria. It most often causes a lung infection, and sometimes it can affect the brain.
Salmonella	Food poisoning	It causes vomiting, diarrhea, and severe stomach upset. It's caused by a non-typhoidal salmonellae bacteria that can be found in the intestinal tracts of animals and humans. The most known method of infection is eating undercooked poultry.
Escherichia coli	Gastrointestinal (GI) distress	The infection may be severe or fatal. This bacteria is most commonly transmitted through contaminated food.
Methicillin-resistant Staphylococcus aureus (MRSA)	Antibiotic-resistant bacteria	Can be deadly, particularly in people who have compromised immune systems. The symptoms include painful abscesses, fever, and inflammation.
Bacterial pneumonia	Lung infection	It's triggered by a number of different bacteria, such as Klebsiella pneumonia, Streptococcus pneumonia, Pseudomonas aeruginosa, etc. They are commonly spread through air particles from sneezing or coughing.
Bacterial vaginosis	Vagina infection	It can cause discharge, itchiness, and painful urination. This is the result of an imbalance in the normal bacterial flora of the vagina.

Clostridium difficile	GI illness	This bacteria is usually located in the intestine. It can cause GI illness when it starts to overgrow due to an impaired immune system or antibiotic use.
Gonorrhea	Sexually Transmitted Infection	The carrier is a bacteria called Neisseria gonorrhoeae. The symptoms are redness and swelling of the infected area, pain, and swelling in testicles, frequency of urination, a persistent sore throat.
Heliobacter pylori	Stomach ulcers and chronic gastritis	The the GI tract may change because of acidity, reflux, smoking, which predisposes to this bacterial infection.

Viral Infections

Viruses are tiny particles of genetic material (RNA or DNA) that are covered with a protein coat. They can't reproduce themselves on their own, so they need to infect organisms to survive. Viruses have a bad rap, though they play a major role in supporting the environment, plants, animals, and humans. For example, some of them serve as protection from other infections. They also help transfer genes among different species in the process of evolution.

We all think of influenza, the common cold, coronavirus, chickenpox, and others when we hear about viruses. Viruses can infect different areas of the body, such as the gastrointestinal, respiratory, and reproductive systems. They can also damage the brain, skin, and liver. Evidence has shown that viruses are often implicated in multiple cancers.

The most common types of viruses are:

- **Rhinovirus** often causes the common cold, but more than 200 different viruses can lead to colds. Cold symptoms like sneezing, coughing, sore throat, and mild headache usually last for up to 2 weeks.
- **Seasonal influenza** is a virus that infects between 5% and 20% of the US population every year. Almost 200,000 people per year need hospitalization due to flu complications. Its symptoms commonly include severe fatigue and body aches.
- **Respiratory Syncytial Virus (RSV)** is a viral infection that causes upper respiratory infections (like colds) and lower respiratory infections like bronchiolitis and pneumonia. It may be very severe in small children, infants, and elderly adults.

Fungal Infections

Fungal infections can be classified as **opportunistic** and **primary**. Opportunistic infections develop mainly in hosts with weak immune system, while primary ones infect immunocompetent hosts.

Opportunistic fungal infections

A lot of fungi are opportunists and are commonly not pathogenic, only if you have a strong immune system, though. Patients who spend more than a week in a hospital can be compromised due to malnutrition, medical procedures, or underlying disorders.

Typical opportunistic systemic fungal infections are:

- candidiasis
- aspergillosis
- mucormycosis
- fusariosis

Primary fungal infections

Primary fungal infections are the result of inhalation of fungal spores, which cause localized pneumonia (primary manifestation of infection). Systemic mycoses commonly have a chronic course. Pneumonia and septicemia with disseminated mycoses are rare diseases and lung lesions progress slowly. It would be months before you discover you are sick due to the absence or lowered severity of symptoms. Sometimes you may experience night sweats, fever, chills, weight loss, anorexia, malaise, and depression. Various organs can be infected and dysfunction. Fungal infections can be **systemic** or **local**.

Local fungal diseases typically infect the skin, mouth (stomatitis), or vagina (candidal vaginitis).

Systemic mycoses that damage highly immunocompromised patients frequently manifest intensely with fungemia and progressive pneumonia.

BEST YOU CAN DO TO AVOID DISEASES

Wash your hands. Washing hands is especially important before eating, before and after preparing food, after using the toilet, and after returning home from being out. Do not touch your nose, mouth, or eyes with your hands, because this is the easiest way for germs to enter your body.

Stay home when ill. Don't go to work or outside if you feel bad, have diarrhea, are vomiting, have chills or a fever. Do, however, go to a doctor if your symptoms persist.

Get vaccinated. Vaccines reduce the chances of contracting diseases.

Prepare food safely. When preparing meals, keep counters and other kitchen surfaces absolutely clean. Cook your food to the proper temperature. For ground meats, the temperature should be at least 160°F, for poultry 165°F, and 145°F for most other meats. Refrigerate leftovers as well — don't allow cooked food to sit at room temperature for a long time.

Don't share personal items. Avoid sharing dining utensils or drinking glasses. Use your own comb, toothbrush, and razor.

Travel wisely. If you like traveling around the world, consult your doctor about special vaccinations, for example, cholera, yellow fever, hepatitis A, typhoid fever.

Practice safe sex. You must always use condoms if you or your partner has or had any sexually transmitted infections.

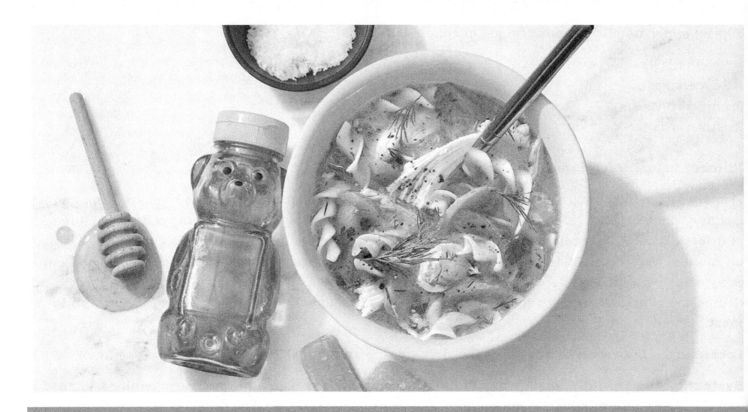

CHAPTER 3. HOW TO STRENGTHEN YOUR IMMUNE SYSTEM

You can protect your body from sniffles and coughing by eating immune-boosting foods.

Best Foods for the Immune System

Oranges are a good source of vitamin C, which helps prevent the common cold. It can also help reduce the severity and duration of a cold.

Blueberries are loaded with antioxidants that prevent and help to treat coughs and colds. Consuming flavonoids — blueberries antioxidants — lowers the chance of catching a cold. Also, it may help fight inflammation.

Apples can help avoid illnesses such as the typical cold. They contain phytochemical antioxidants that reduce the chances of chronic diseases and help boost immunity.

Red Peppers is also a rich source of vitamin C. According to Harvard Health Letter review, 200 ml of vitamin C every day helps make the duration of symptoms shorter by 14% in children and 8% in adults.

Spinach is packed with vitamin C and loaded with digestion-regulating fiber.

Mushrooms increase the strength of immunity-boosting T-cells. They also reduce inflammatory-inducing proteins.

Miso. Being made from soy, miso is loaded with isoflavone antioxidants that boost immunity and reduce inflammation.

Ginger decreases inflammation,. It stores heat in the form of gingerol, a close relative of capsaicin. It may help reduce and ease chronic pain and possess cholesterol-lowering properties.

Garlic can help slow down the hardening of the arteries and lower blood pressure. The immune-boosting effects of garlic is derived from a large concentration of sulfur-containing compounds, such as allicin.

Turmeric. This spice contains curcumin, a strong anti-inflammatory compound. Curcumin triggers the production of T-cells.

Poultry. Both turkey and chicken are rich in Vitamin B6. It plays a huge role in many of the chemical reactions that occur in our bodies and is necessary for the formation of new red blood cells. Broth cooked by boiling chicken bones includes chondroitin, gelatin, and other nutrients for gut health and immunity.

Wild Salmon and Light White Tuna are loaded with zinc.

Green Tea contains flavonoids that boost immunity and has anti-inflammatory affects. It also includes the antioxidant catechin, which is known to be a strong antiviral and antibacterial.

Greek Yogurt is rich in probiotics and contains more protein than usual yogurt.

Raw Honey is helpful in ease pain in sore and itchy throats. Honey also acts as an antibacterial, killing any microbes in the body that can cause you to get sick.

Worst Foods for the Immune System

Sugary Snacks. Refined sugars can suppress the immune system. Refined sugar targets and attacks the cells that fight against bacteria. After you eat something sugary, the effect can continue for hours.

Soda. If you like drinking soda — it doesn't matter what sweetener has been used — you're harming your immune system. Even diet soda is a bad option. Soda doesn't have any beneficial nutrients, so drinkers can't get enough calcium, magnesium, and vitamin A — all essential elements for the immune system. And phosphoric acid can deplete magnesium and calcium in the body.

Fried Foods are full of fats that can increase the amount of bad cholesterol and inflammation in the body. In addition, it accumulates acrylamide — a dangerous carcinogen.

Processed Foods contain a hefty amount of refined sugar, hidden flavorings, and carbohydrates. Even cereal and bread, organically processed foods, may contain immune-suppressing sugar.

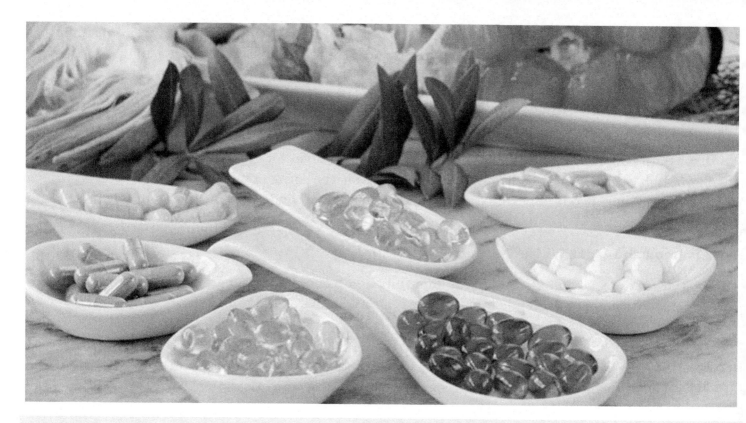

ESSENTIAL NUTRIENTS FOR THE IMMUNE SYSTEM

Good nutrition is essential if you want to strengthen your immune system, which should protect us from seasonal illness and other diseases. No one supplement or food can totally prevent illness, but you can try to include vitamins and minerals that are important for our immune system in your overall eating plan on a regular basis.

Vitamins, Minerals & Proteins

Vitamin A

Vitamin A supports the cells' structure in the respiratory tract, skin, and gut We need vitamin A to produce antibodies that neutralize harmful and infected pathogens.

You can find Vitamin A in egg yolks, oily fish, tofu, cheese, seeds, nuts, legumes, and whole grains. In addition, vegetables include beta-carotene, which our body converts into vitamin A. Beta-carotene can be found in leafy greens and yellow, orange vegetables such as pumpkin and carrots.

B vitamins

B vitamins, specifically B6, B9, and B12, help your body respond once it has recognized hostile microbes. They influence the activity and production of killer cells. These cells work by causing infected cells to become expose (this process is called apoptosis).

B6	legumes, cereals, fruit, green leafy vegetables, nuts, chicken, fish, meat
B9 (folate)	green leafy vegetables, legumes, nuts, and seeds
B12 (cyanocobalamin)	eggs, meat and dairy, fortified soy milk

Vitamins C and E

When your body is fighting an infection, it is called oxidative stress. It causes the production of free radicals that can damage cell walls, exacerbating inflammation. Vitamins C and E can help protect cells from this process. Vitamin C also participates in cleaning up the cellular mess by producing special cells, such as lymphocytes, neutrophils, and phagocytes, to mount an immune response.

Oranges, limes, lemons, kiwifruit, berries, tomatoes, broccoli, and capsicum are rich in vitamin C. Vitamin E can be found in vegetable oils, green leafy vegetables, and nuts.

Vitamin D

Particular cells require vitamin D to destroy pathogens that trigger infection. For a majority of people, it's enough to spend only a few minutes outside, while others need to take supplements. Vitamin D supplements may help protect our body from acute respiratory infections. You can also get this vitamin from products such as eggs, fish, and some milks.

Iron

Iron participates in killing pathogens – it increases the number of free radicals that destroy microbes. Iron also controls enzyme reactions needed for immune cells to detect and target pathogens. The greatest source of iron is whole-grain foods, meat, chicken and fish, legumes.

Zinc

Zinc helps build up the mucous membranes and integrity of the skin. Zinc function as an antioxidant – it helps clean the damage caused by oxidative stress. You can find this mineral in seafood, chicken, meat, dried beans, nuts.

Selenium

Selenium, like zink, eliminates the consequences of oxidative stress. Find it in meat, nuts (especially Brazil nuts), cereals, and mushrooms.

Protein

Protein is very important for our body and immune system, especially for recovery and healing processes. Find protein in lean meat, seafood, poultry, eggs, soy products, beans and peas, unsalted nuts and seeds.

Omega-3 Fatty Acids

They are that type of essential fatty acid that helps to keep the immune system's ability to recognize pathogens and suppress inflammation. The main source is oily fish (mackerel, salmon, tuna, herring sardines, trout), walnuts, flaxseed, chia seeds.

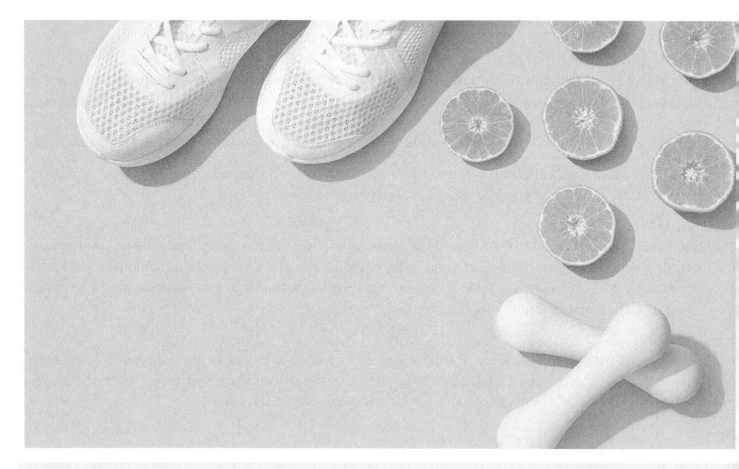

WHY YOU NEED TO HAVE AN ACTIVE AND HEALTHY LIFESTYLE

The idea of boosting the immune system is exciting, but it's not so easy to do it. You should realize that the immunity is not a single entity — it's a system. If you want it to function correctly, you need to maintain balance and harmony in your body. The researchers don't know exactly how to work all immune systems interconnectedness and intricacies. For now, there has been no clinically established a direct correlation between lifestyle and improved immune function.

Don't think that your lifestyle doesn't affect your immunity, and you don't need to look after yourself at all. General healthy-living strategies are an excellent start to strengthen your immune system.

The Importance of Exercises

Regular physical activity is a necessary aspect of strengthening our immune system and managing stress. The scientists found out that active people who engage in regular physical activity are less exposed to infectious diseases than sedentary and inactivity ones. Also, your physically active lifestyle may lower the chance of chronic diseases, which could make your immune system weaker, such as diabetes, cardiovascular disease, and obesity.

How does it work? Physical activity helps to flush bacteria out of the lungs, reducing your chances of catching a cold, flu, or other diseases. Exercise also relieves levels of stress hormones, including cortisol and adrenaline. Lower levels of these hormones might help to protect your body against illness.

Exercise also helps decrease your risk of getting a heart disease. It keeps bones strong and healthy. There are few theories about the effect of exercise on the immune system, though none of them have been proven:

- Exercise leads to changes in white blood cells and antibodies. They begin to circulate faster, so they will recognize illnesses earlier than they did it before.
- During and right after exercise, the body temperature rises for a short period of time that may help fight infection and bacteria before it grows up. This phenomenon is close to the process when you have a fever.

Though exercise can make your life better, you shouldn't overdo it. If you already exercise, carry on like that, you don't need to exercise more because it may only hurt you. Long-term and heavy training like intense gym workouts or marathon, can cause harm to your body.

Plan your own moderate program to increase your physical activity. It can include:

- bicycling a few times a week
- going to the gym every day
- taking daily 20 to 30-minute walks

It will make you feel more energetic and healthier. So go and take an aerobics class or go for t walk. If you don't want to go outside, try to do it at home. For a cardio workout, do jumping jacks, then high knees, butt kicks, burpees, and switch jumps for 15 seconds each. Repeat the circuit 5-10 times, depending on how much you can do.

Regular exercise is one of the first steps to healthy living and strong immunity. It improves blood pressure and cardiovascular health, control body weight, and prevent a huge variety of diseases. It works as a healthy diet – it contributes to general good health and then to a healthy immune system.

Healthy and Unhealthy Habits

Be sure, a healthy lifestyle will help to build up your immune system, but it includes more than just regular exercises. Following the general recommendations for good health is the best measure you may take to actually maintain the immune system active and balanced. Each part of your body and the immune system isn't an exception, functions better when it's protected from environmental assaults, and you're guided by wisdom and healthy habits like these:

- maintain a healthy weight
- diet high in vegetables and fruits
- don't smoke
- drink alcohol only in moderation
- get enough sleep

- exercise regularly
- wash your hands frequently
- cook meats thoroughly
- minimize the stress
- get used to a healthy diet

Few words about the last habit. A healthy diet is a basement for the immune system's strength. To run properly, the immune system needs regular and quality nourishment. So, one of the keys to a healthy life and disease invulnerability is a well-balanced diet.

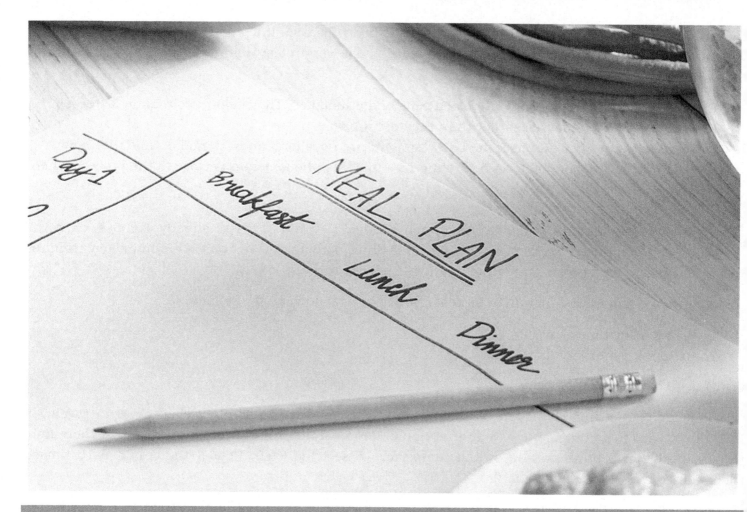

CHAPTER 4. 14-DAY MEAL PLAN TO RECOVERY YOUR IMMUNE SYSTEM

Eating healthy food is an important part of building up your immune system.

■ **Eat only as much as you need**

At the end of a meal, you may feel satisfied, but not stuffed. Stick to healthy lunches and dinners, and once a week, you can reward yourself with your favorite meal.

■ **Eat smaller portions**

If you serve meals in a smaller bowl or on plates, you can make your brain think it's a large portion. You can also add to your meal with leafy greens or fruits/vegetables.

■ **Don't think about limits**

When you forbid yourself certain foods, you will want them more. Reduce your portion sizes of unhealthy food and don't eat them frequently. Eventually, you may find you want them less.

■ **Limit your snacks**

Do not overestimate your willpower, and reduce the amount of unhealthy snacks in your home or get rid of them entirely. Fill your kitchen with healthy snacks such as fresh crunchy vegetables with hummus and fruit.

■ **Control your emotions when eating**

Learn healthier ways to release your stress and emotions, and there won't be any difficulties with overeating.

■ Avoid eating late at night

The best time to eat your dinner is 14-16 hours before breakfast the next morning. Research shows that eating food in the most active period of the day and giving the digestive system a long break can help to control your body weight.

■ Add more vegetables and fruit to your meals

Fruit and vegetables are nutritious and low in calories and are loaded with antioxidants, minerals, vitamins, and fiber.

■ Plan your meals

Choose healthy recipes that you can enjoy and build your diet around them. Plan your meals at the start of each week, so there's no room to eat poorly.

■ Find quality foods

Look for fresh fruit and vegetables, fish and poultry, dairy products and whole-grain bread.

Focusing on essential nutrition is the first step in strengthening your immune system. The main task of this book was creating of 14-Day Recover Meal Plan that will help you to make your daily ration much healthier than before. It's called "recovery" because the nutrients you will get during the next two weeks may help you to recover the protective functions of your body and make up the lack of all vitamins and minerals that are required for the immune system proper work.

Its recovery plan was tested by author and his friend who was suffering from seasonal colds for last two years. This book guided him during two weeks and he changed his lifestyle and eating habits. After two weeks, he's still following these recommendations and became not only less exposed to seasonal diseases, but also has a permanent weight now. He was asked what helped him most of all this book and the answer was meal plan and exercises. "Before this meal plan I was eating a lot of garbage food that I liked and often skipped breakfast or lunch, so snacks as chips or other junk food were always ready to hand. Never thought before that my ration was one of the reasons of these colds!", he said, "So after changing my diet, the next step was exercising. I became more active and refused from my sedentary lifestyle. I'm still amazed by how these changes improved my life!".

This plan is based on recipes rich in fruits and vegetables. They will help you to get vitamin A, vitamin C, vitamin E, folate, and copper. Eating animal and plant-based proteins loaded with minerals and vitamins such as iron, vitamin D, vitamin B6, B12 is also part of the plan. Support your gut with pre- and probiotics that you can find in fibrous food and probiotics fermented foods, like yogurt.

Your diet will be diversified with delicious and nutritious drink and dishes to avoid any discomfort from the same meal every day. Such combination of recipes was selected to get maximum health benefits. Some days will include snacks to get more nutrients during the day and hot tea that will help to boost your immunity, some days won't – they are discharge day. If you're sure that this plan will work for you, it's time to start! Remember, everyone is unique, so listen to your body!

REMEMBER! *BEFORE START ANY DIET CONSULT THE DOCTOR OR NUTRITIONIST FIRST!*

DAY 1

Breakfast	Salmon Toasts with Scrambled Eggs (p. 34)
Snack 1	Coconut Milk Yogurt (p. 30)
Lunch	Tandoori Salmon with Toasted Greens (p. 80)
Snack 2	Vitamin C Bites (p. 72)
Dinner	Roasted Chicken Soup (p. 85)
Tea Time	Ginger Lemon Tea (p. 99)

DAY 2

Breakfast	Whole Grain Fruity Bowl (p. 36)
Snack 1	Thyme Roasted Almonds (p. 68)
Lunch	Buddha Rice Bowl with Tahini Dressing (p. 60)
Snack 2	1 Avocado + Crackers
Dinner	Tandoori Salmon with Toasted Greens (p. 80)

DAY 3

Breakfast	Mango Granola with Yogurt (p. 35)
Snack 1	Pumpkin Seed Bars (p. 87)
Lunch	Spring Vegetable Chicken Soup (p. 57)
Snack 2	Fall Salad (p. 63)
Dinner	Buddha Rice Bowl with Tahini Dressing (p. 60)
Dessert	Goji Berry Bowl (p. 93)

DAY 4

Breakfast	Spinach, Feta, and Pepper Omelet (p. 32)
Snack 1	Salmon Avocado Toast (p. 75)
Lunch	Pistachio Buddha Bowl (p. 62)
Snack 2	Unsalted Nuts
Dinner	Kale, Beet and Tuna Salad (p. 66)
Tea Time	Herbal Tea (p. 94)

DAY 5

Breakfast	Mango Kiwi Breakfast Bowl (p. 29) Grapefruit Pear Smoothie (p. 38)
Snack 1	Winter Citrus Salad (p. 73)
Lunch	Vegetable Ramen (p. 50)
Snack 2	1 Avocado + Crackers
Dinner	Tuna Potato Plate (p. 81)
Tea Time	Herbal Tea (p. 94)

DAY 6

Breakfast	Vegetable Latkes (p. 31) Turkey Apple Sausage with Sage (p. 33)
Snack 1	1 Whole-Wheat bread slice + 1 Tbsp peanut butter
Lunch	Broccoli Asparagus Rice (p. 58) 2 Salmon Avocado Toasts (p. 75)
Dinner	Tuna Pita Pockets (p. 69)

DAY 7

Breakfast	4-5 Whole Wheat Pancakes (p. 37)
Lunch	Garlic Pasta (p. 54)
Dinner	Grilled Spiced Chicken (p. 84) Watermelon Green Salad (p. 70)
Dessert	Turmeric Chia Pudding (p. 89)

DAY 8

Breakfast	Mango Granola with Yogurt (p. 35)
Snack 1	Fruit Custard (p. 88)
Lunch	Miso Soup (p. 52)
Snack 2	Orange Chicken Salad (p. 65)
Dinner	Eastern Tuna Steak (p. 78) Fall Salad (p. 63)
Tea Time	Mandarin Herb Tea (p. 95)

DAY 9

Breakfast	Whole Grain Fruity Bowl (p. 36)
Snack 1	Lemon Ginger Bites (p. 64)
Lunch	Miso Soup (p. 52)
Snack 2	1 Avocado + Crackers
Dinner	Grilled Spiced Chicken (p. 84) Lemon Ginger Stir-Fry (p. 79)

DAY 10

Breakfast	Mango Granola with Yogurt (p. 35)
Snack 1	Pumpkin Seed Bars (p. 87)
Lunch	Mustard Glazed Salmon and Zoodles (p. 51)
Snack 2	Lemon Ginger Bites (p. 64)
Dinner	Pistachio Buddha Bowl (p. 62)
Dessert	Apple Tart (p. 91) Ginger Lemon Tea (p. 99)

DAY 11

Breakfast	Spinach, Feta, and Pepper Omelet (p. 32)
Snack 1	Pumpkin Seed Bars (p. 87)
Lunch	Pistachio Buddha Bowl (p. 62)
Snack 2	Lemon Ginger Bites (p. 64)
Dinner	Kale, Beet and Tuna Salad (p. 66)
Tea Time	Herbal Tea (p. 94)

DAY 12

Breakfast	Whole Grain Fruity Bowl (p. 36) Grapefruit Mango Smoothie (p. 47)
Snack 1	Pumpkin Seed Bars (p. 87)
Lunch	Kale Mushroom Soup (p. 49)
Snack 2	1 Avocado + Crackers
Dinner	Potatoes and Green Beans with Tuna Steak (p. 53)
Tea Time	Herbal Tea (p. 94)

DAY 13

Breakfast	Salmon Toasts with Scrambled Eggs (p. 34)
Snack 1	Thyme Roasted Almonds (p. 68)
Lunch	Kale Mushroom Soup (p. 49)
Dinner	Mung Dal (p. 77)
Tea Time	Ginger Lemon Tea (p. 99)

DAY 14

Breakfast	Spinach, Feta, and Peppers Omelet (p. 32)
Lunch	Garlic Pasta (p. 54)
Dinner	Grilled Spiced Chicken (p. 84) Sprouts (p. 59)
Dessert	Baked Apples (p. 92)

MANGO KIWI BREAKFAST BOWL

SERVINGS: 1   PREP TIME: 5 min.   COOK TIME: 5 min.

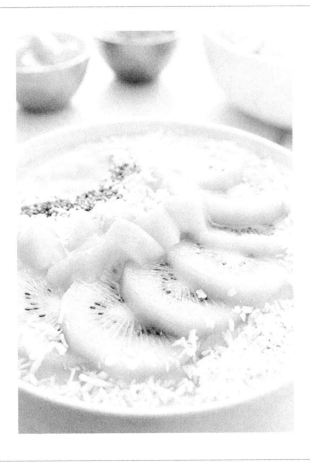

CARBS – 44 g   FAT – 5 g   PROTEIN – 12 g   CALORIES – 257

Ingredients

- *1 cup dairy-free coconut yogurt*
- *1 kiwi, sliced*
- *1 tsp pure maple syrup*
- *½ mango, diced*
- *1 Tbsp chia seeds*
- *1 Tbsp coconut flakes*

Directions

1. Combine maple syrup and yogurt in a bowl.
2. Top with kiwi and mango.
3. Sprinkle with chia seeds and coconut flakes.
4. Enjoy!

COCONUT MILK YOGURT

SERVINGS: 4   PREP TIME: 1 day   COOK TIME: 1 day

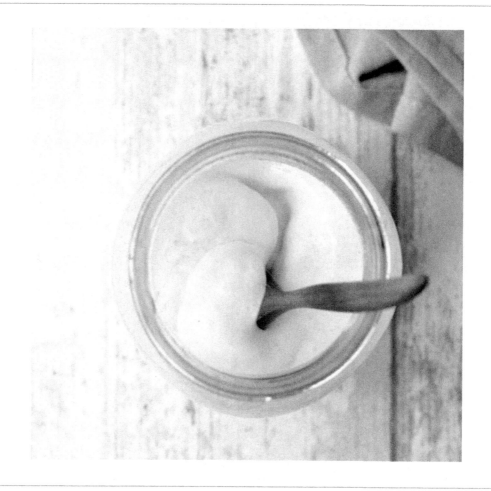

CARBS – 10 g   FAT – 7 g   PROTEIN – 1 g   CALORIES – 110

Ingredients

- *1 (14-oz) can full-fat coconut milk*
- *2 probiotic capsules*
- *½ tsp pure maple syrup*
- *⅛ tsp sea salt*

Directions

1. Sterilize a mason jar and lid by submerging it in boiling water for 10 minutes. Take out and drain it. Set aside.
2. Pour all coconut milk in the mason jar and shake to mix.
3. Add the contents of probiotic capsules to the jar. Shake well.
4. Cover with lid and let it sit for 1-2 days to activate the fermentation process. Shake it from time to time.
5. After 24-48 hours, put the mason jar into the refrigerator.
6. Serve your portion with maple syrup and sea salt.
7. Keep in the fridge for 7 days. Enjoy!

VEGETABLE LATKES

SERVINGS: 1   PREP TIME: 10 min.   COOK TIME: 20 min.

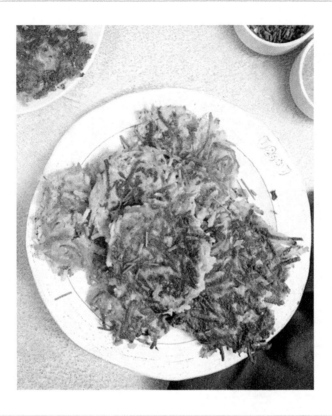

CARBS – 15 g   FAT – 20 g   PROTEIN – 10 g   CALORIES – 268

Ingredients

- *1 cup daikon radish, shredded*
- *1 cup zucchini, shredded*
- *1 cup carrot, shredded*
- *1 cup white sweet potato, shredded*
- *1½ scoops collagen peptides*
- *2 Tbsp almond flour*
- *½ tsp garlic powder*
- *½ tsp salt*
- *¼ tsp black pepper*
- *2 medium eggs*
- *¼ cup avocado oil*

Directions

1. Preheat oven to 400°F.
2. Line a rimmed baking sheet with parchment paper.
3. Place a skillet in the oven to heat for 5 minutes.
4. Squeeze the vegetables to remove excess water and add all ingredients (except oil) to a large bowl.
5. Mix well and let rest for 5-10 minutes.
6. Heat the oil in the skillet over medium-high.
7. Add a scoop of vegetable mixture to the pan and flatten it into a patty. Cook for 1-2 minutes each side.
8. Repeat with remaining mixture.
9. Transfer cooked patties to the prepared sheet pan and bake 10-12 minutes.
10. Remove from oven and let cool.
11. Serve with your favorite sauce. Enjoy!

SPINACH, FETA, AND PEPPERS OMELET

SERVINGS: 1   PREP TIME: 10 min.   COOK TIME: 10 min.

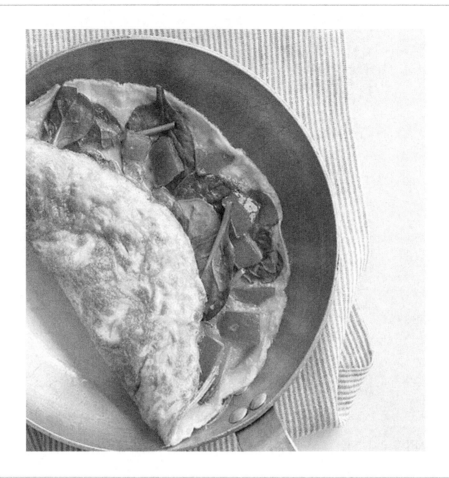

CARBS – 9 g   FAT – 31 g   PROTEIN – 19 g   CALORIES – 398

Ingredients

- *2 eggs*
- *2 Tbsp half-and-half*
- *⅛ tsp garlic powder*
- *½ cup bell peppers, chopped*
- *1 cup spinach*
- *¼ cup crumbled feta cheese*
- *2 Tbsp butter , divided*
- *Salt and pepper, to taste*

Directions

1. Whisk eggs and half-and-half in a bowl.
2. Add salt and pepper. Set aside.
3. Heat 1 Tbsp butter in a pan.
4. Add peppers and saute for 5 minutes.
5. Add spinach, salt, pepper, garlic powder. Cook for 2 minutes, stirring.
6. Transfer vegetables to a bowl and wipe the pan with a paper towel.
7. Heat 1 Tbsp butter over medium heat.
8. Add eggs, and after 1 minute, start to pull them to the center from sides.
9. Continue until the omelet is almost cooked (you will see a layer of unset eggs on top).
10. Add veggies and cheese to one half of omelet.
11. Fold in half using a spatula. Enjoy!

TURKEY APPLE SAUSAGE WITH SAGE

SERVINGS: 8   PREP TIME: 10 min.   COOK TIME: 10 min.

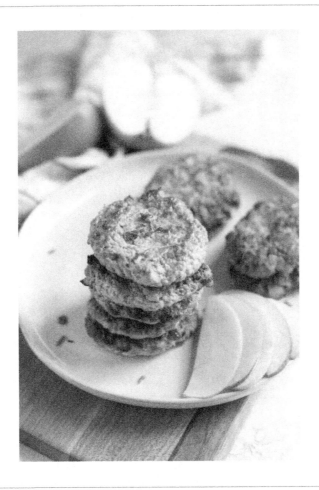

CARBS – 6 g   FAT – 5 g   PROTEIN – 12 g   CALORIES – 110

Ingredients

- 1 lb organic ground turkey
- 1 large apple, shredded
- 4 Tbsp chopped fresh sage
- 2 cloves garlic, crushed
- 2½ Tbsp fennel
- 1½ tsp fresh thyme
- ½ tsp sea salt
- 1½ Tbsp ground pepper
- 1 apple, sliced

Directions

1. Mix all ingredients in a bowl.
2. Make 8 small patties from the mixture.
3. Heat the skillet over medium heat.
4. Add patties to the skillet, cover with the lid.
5. Cook for 5-7 minutes, until they're cooked.
6. Serve with sliced apples.
7. Enjoy!

SALMON TOAST WITH SCRAMBLED EGGS

SERVINGS: 1   PREP TIME: 20 min.   COOK TIME: 5 min.

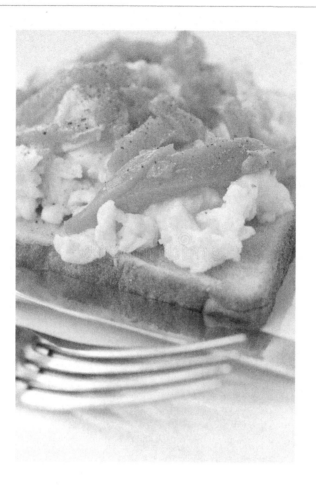

CARBS – 17 g   FAT – 44 g   PROTEIN – 33 g   CALORIES – 605

Ingredients

- *1 Tbsp butter*
- *2 large eggs*
- *1 Tbsp milk*
- *1 slice wholemeal bread, toasted*
- *2 slices smoked or fresh salmon*
- *Salt and freshly ground black pepper, to taste + more black pepper for serving*

Directions

1. Melt butter in a saucepan on low heat.
2. Add eggs, stirring constantly.
3. Cook eggs for 4-5 minutes(they should be creamy).
4. When they start to get thick, add milk.
5. Remove from heat .
6. Put bread slices on a plate.
7. Place scrambled eggs on toast and put salmon slices over the eggs.
8. Sprinkle with black pepper.
9. Enjoy!

MANGO GRANOLA WITH YOGURT

SERVINGS: 4   PREP TIME: 10 min.   COOK TIME: 30 min.

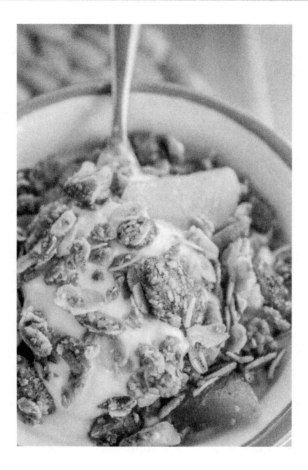

CARBS – 53 g   FAT – 15 g   PROTEIN – 26 g   CALORIES – 423

Ingredients

- ¼ cup canola oil
- ¼ cup agave syrup
- ¼ cup clover honey
- 1 tsp ground cinnamon
- 2 Tbsp packed light brown sugar
- 1 tsp vanilla extract
- 3 cups old-fashioned rolled oats
- ¾ cup slivered almonds
- ½ cup raw sunflower seeds
- ½ cup raw pumpkin seeds
- 2 Tbsp flax seeds
- 2 Tbsp wheat germ
- ¼ tsp salt
- 1 cup diced dried sweetened mango
- 1 pint 2% Greek yogurt

Directions

1. Preheat the oven to 325°F.
2. Line a rimmed baking sheet with parchment paper.
3. Mix honey, agave syrup, canola oil, vanilla extract, cinnamon, and brown sugar in a small bowl.
4. Combine the oats, almonds, sunflower seeds, pumpkin seeds, flax seeds, wheat germ, salt in another bowl.
5. Mix wet and dry mixtures, stirring well.
6. Spread mixture on the baking sheet evenly.
7. Bake for 25-30 minutes, until crisp and browned. Stir occasionally.
8. Remove from the oven and let cool.
9. Mix granola with mango and serve with yogurt. Enjoy!

WHOLE GRAIN FRUITY BOWL

SERVINGS: 2   PREP TIME: 5 min.   COOK TIME: 5 min.

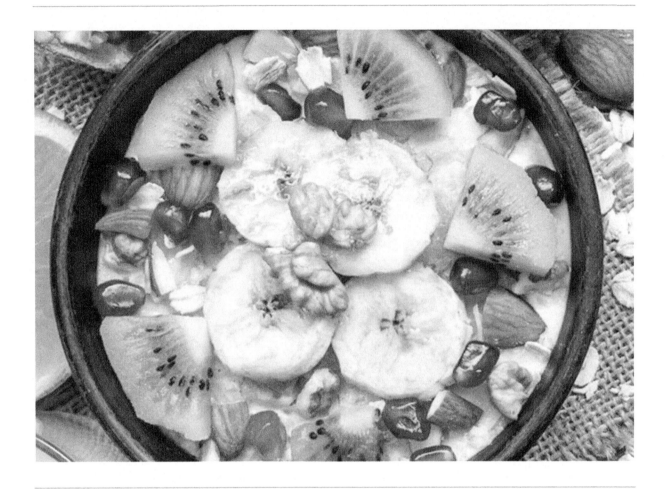

CARBS – 52 g   FAT – 12 g   PROTEIN – 10 g   CALORIES – 338

Ingredients

- ½ cup whole grain (wheat farina)
- ½ cup white corn grits
- 1 cup vanilla almond milk
- 1 cup water
- 2 Tbsp pure maple syrup
- 1 tsp pure vanilla extract
- ½ tsp ground ginger
- ¼ tsp sea salt
- 2 kiwis, sliced
- 1 banana, thinly sliced
- ½ cup pomegranate seeds
- ¼ cup chopped walnuts

Directions

1. Add almond milk, water, maple syrup, vanilla, ginger, and salt to a pot. Mix well.
2. Bring it to simmer.
3. Add farina and grits. Bring to a low boil.
4. Cover with lid. Turn the heat to low and let it simmer for 5 minutes, until cereal starts to thicken.
5. Divide the cereal between 2 bowls.
6. Top each bowl with kiwis, banana, pomegranate seeds, and walnuts.
7. Enjoy!

WHOLE WHEAT PANCAKES

SERVINGS: 10   PREP TIME: 10 min.   COOK TIME: 20 min.

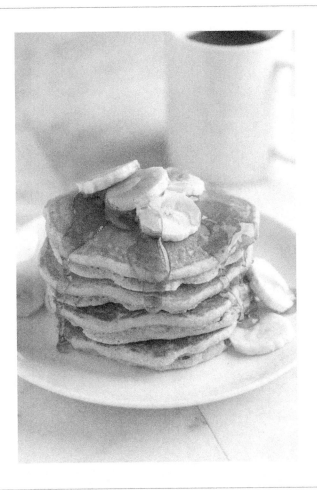

CARBS – 10 g   FAT – 4 g   PROTEIN – 4 g   CALORIES – 87

Ingredients

- *1 cup white whole wheat flour*
- *6 Tbsp buttermilk powder*
- *¼ cup ground flaxseed*
- *1 tsp baking powder*
- *1 tsp baking soda*
- *½ tsp ground cinnamon*
- *Pinch of salt*
- *1 egg*
- *1½ cups water*
- *2 Tbsp canola oil*

Directions

1. Combine flour, buttermilk powder, flaxseed, baking powder, baking soda, cinnamon, salt in a bowl. Stir well.
2. Whisk egg in another bowl, then add water and oil, and whisk again.
3. Add flour mixture to the egg and whisk until well combined.
4. Let it rest for 5 minutes.
5. Preheat a griddle over medium heat and grease with cooking spray.
6. Put ¼ cup pancake batter on the griddle.
7. Cook for 1-2 minutes until it's brown and bubbling on top.
8. Flip and cook for 2 minutes.
9. Repeat for the remaining batter.
10. Serve with your favorite toppings.
11. Enjoy!

GRAPEFRUIT PEAR SMOOTHIE

SERVINGS: 2   PREP TIME: 10 min.   COOK TIME: 10 min.

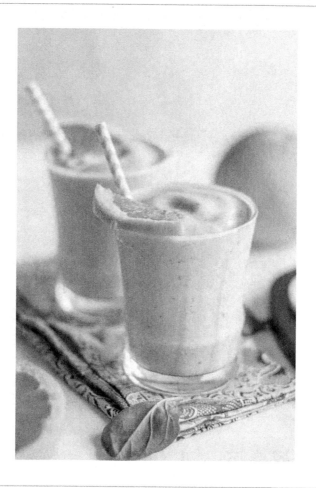

CARBS – 27 g   FAT – 0 g   PROTEIN – 2 g   CALORIES – 108

Ingredients

- *1 pear, chopped*
- *1 orange, chopped*
- *1 grapefruit, chopped*
- *1 piece ginger, chopped*
- *1 large handful spinach*
- *½ cup water*

Directions

1. Blend the spinach with the water.
2. Then add the remaining ingredients to the blender.
3. Blend until smooth.
4. Divide evenly between 2 glasses.
5. Enjoy!

CINNAMON CITRUS JUICE

SERVINGS: 2   PREP TIME: 5 min.   COOK TIME: 5 min.

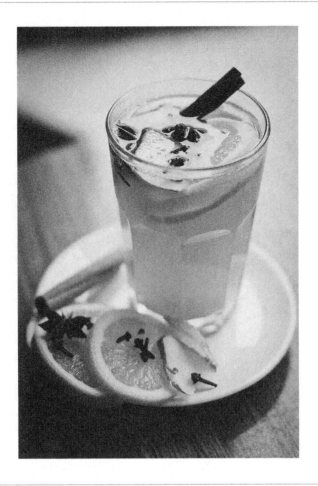

CARBS – 27 g   FAT – 0 g   PROTEIN – 2 g   CALORIES – 120

Ingredients

- *6 oranges, peeled and chopped*
- *2 lemons, peeled and chopped*
- *1 thumb fresh ginger, peeled*
- *2 large carrots, peeled and chopped*
- *2 tsp cinnamon*
- *¼ cup water*
- *1 tsp honey*
- *4-6 ice cubes*
- *2 cinnamon sticks*

Directions

1. Add all ingredients (except ice, cinnamon sticks, and lemon) to the blender.
2. Blend until smooth (20-25 seconds).
3. Strain the juice into a jug.
4. Add ice, lemon, and cinnamon sticks to a glass and pour in the juice.
5. Enjoy!

BERRY TURMERIC SMOOTHIE

SERVINGS: 2   PREP TIME: 5 min.   COOK TIME: 5 min.

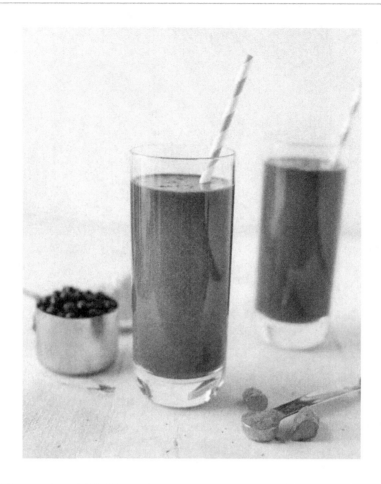

CARBS – 27 g   FAT – 2 g   PROTEIN – 8 g   CALORIES – 151

Ingredients

- ¾ cup unsweetened vanilla almond milk
- 2 cups baby spinach
- ½ cup nonfat plain Greek yogurt
- 3 Tbsp old-fashioned rolled oats
- 1½ cups frozen mixed berries
- ½ tsp ground turmeric
- ¼ tsp ground ginger
- 2-3 tsp honey

Directions

1. Add ingredients to the blender in this order: almond milk, spinach, yogurt, oats, berries, turmeric, ginger, honey.
2. Blend until smooth.
3. Enjoy!

GREEN CUCUMBER MINT SMOOTHIE

SERVINGS: 2   PREP TIME: 5 min.   COOK TIME: 5 min.

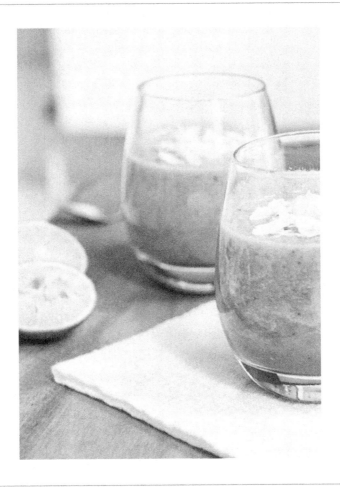

CARBS – 22 g   FAT – 2 g   PROTEIN – 4 g   CALORIES – 105

Ingredients

- *1½ oz collard greens*
- *1 pear, chopped*
- *2 mini cucumbers, chopped*
- *1 bunch mint, stemmed*
- *1 lime, juiced*
- *1 tbsp chia seeds*
- *1 cup water*
- *1 cup ice*

Directions

1. Mix water and greens in a blender.
2. Blend for 30 seconds.
3. Add rest ingredients to the smoothie.
4. Blend for 30 seconds .
5. Enjoy!

CARROT GINGER CITRUS SMOOTHIE

SERVINGS: 2   PREP TIME: 5 min.   COOK TIME: 5 min.

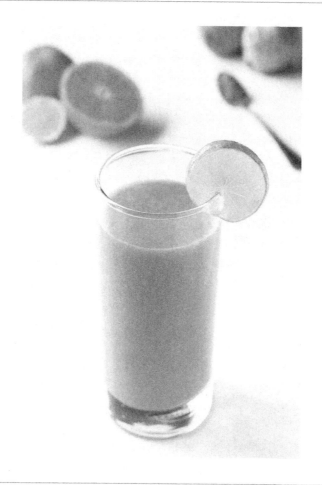

CARBS – 32 g   FAT – 11 g   PROTEIN – 10 g   CALORIES – 251

Ingredients

- *3 mandarins*
- *1 thin slice lemon, skin on*
- *2 carrots, chopped*
- *1 banana, sliced into chunks*
- *1-inch knob fresh ginger, pilled*
- *3 tbs hemp hearts*
- *½ tsp ground turmeric*
- *1 cup water*

Directions

1. Add mandarin, lemon, carrots, banana, ginger, hemp hearts, turmeric, and water to the blender.
2. Start slow, then increase speed up to high until it's smooth (45 seconds).
3. Serve with lemon slice.
4. Enjoy!

SPINACH MANGO SMOOTHIE

SERVINGS: 2   PREP TIME: 5 min.   COOK TIME: 5 min.

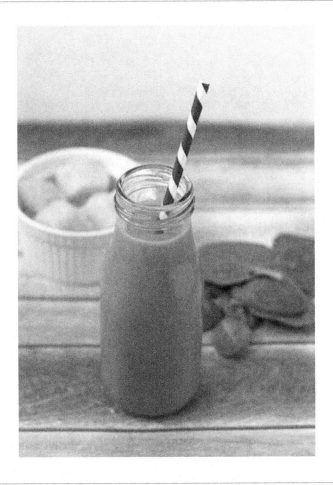

CARBS – 35 g   FAT – 7 g   PROTEIN – 18 g   CALORIES – 276

Ingredients

- 1½ cups spinach
- ¼ cup celery
- ¼ cup parsley fresh
- 2 cups water
- 1 cucumber, peeled
- ½ inch ginger
- 3 cups mango, frozen
- 1 lemon, peeled and seeded

Directions

1. Blend all green ingredients with water.
2. Add remaining ingredients and blend until smooth.
3. Enjoy!

SPINACH KALE SMOOTHIE

SERVINGS: 1   PREP TIME: 5 min.   COOK TIME: 5 min.

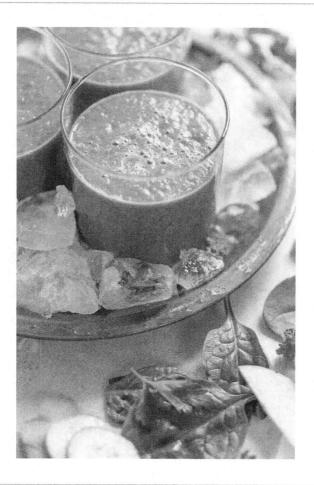

CARBS – 82 g   FAT – 8 g   PROTEIN – 17 g   CALORIES – 175

Ingredients

- *1 cup baby spinach*
- *1 leaf curly kale, stem removed*
- *1 medium rib celery*
- *1 medium cucumber, peeled and chopped*
- *1-inch fresh ginger root, peeled*
- *1 lime juiced*
- *Pinch sea salt*
- *1 cup ice*

Directions

1. Add spinach, kale, celery, cucumber, ginger, lime juice, sea salt to a blender.
2. Add ice and blend until smooth.
3. Pour into a glass.
4. Enjoy!

ORANGE CARROT GINGER JUICE

SERVINGS: 2   PREP TIME: 10 min.   COOK TIME: 10 min.

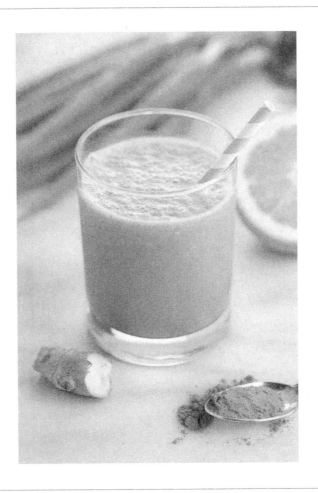

CARBS – 69 g   FAT – 1 g   PROTEIN – 5 g   CALORIES – 273

Ingredients

- *7 oranges, halved*
- *4 carrots, chopped*
- *2.5-inch fresh ginger, peeled and chopped*

Directions

1. Add all the ingredients to the blender. If using a juicer, follow its instructions
2. Blend for 1 minute, then strain the juice.
3. Pour into glasses.
4. Enjoy!

GINGER LEMONADE

SERVINGS: 2   PREP TIME: 5 min.   COOK TIME: 5 min.

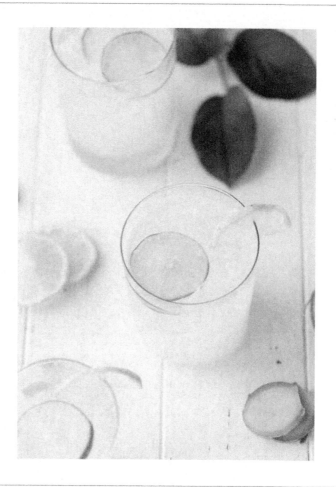

CARBS – 36 g   FAT – 0 g   PROTEIN – 0 g   CALORIES – 140

Ingredients

- *1 medium organic lemon, peeled and sliced*
- *Zest of 1 lemon*
- *10 g fresh ginger, peeled and sliced*
- *2 Tbsp honey*
- *2 cups (500 ml) warm water*

Directions

1. Place all the ingredients in the blender and blend until smooth, 1-2 minutes.
2. Strain the juice and pout into glasses.
3. Enjoy!

GRAPEFRUIT MANGO SMOOTHIE

SERVINGS: 2   PREP TIME: 5 min.   COOK TIME: 5 min.

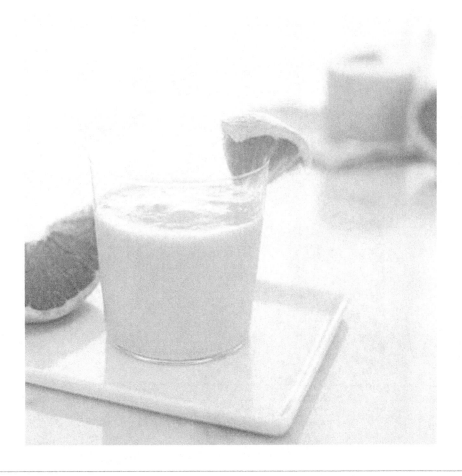

CARBS – 32 g   FAT – 4 g   PROTEIN – 8 g   CALORIES – 184

Ingredients

- 1 wintersweet grapefruit, segmented
- 1 cup frozen mango chunks
- ½ cup plain greek yogurt
- ½ cup milk of choice
- ½ tsp grated fresh ginger
- ¼ tsp turmeric powder
- 1 tsp honey

Directions

1. Blend all ingredients until smooth.
2. Pour into a glass
3. Enjoy!

CHICKEN WONTON SOUP

SERVINGS: 4 PREP TIME: 10 min. COOK TIME: 15 min.

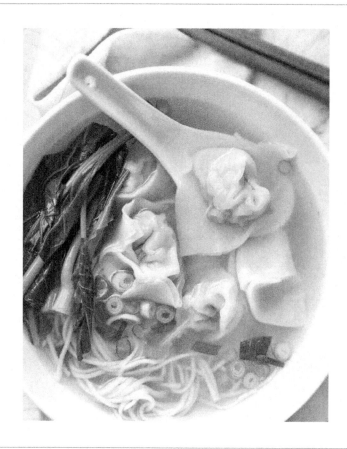

CARBS – 16 g FAT – 2 g PROTEIN – 8 g CALORIES – 120

Ingredients

- *1 Tbsp coconut oil*
- *3 cloves garlic, minced*
- *1 yellow onion, sliced*
- *32 oz bone broth*
- *¼ cup coconut aminos*
- *½ lb frozen wontons*
- *¼ lb rice noodles*
- *½ lb cooked chicken breast, shredded*
- *Juice of 1 lime*
- *2 Tbsp red pepper flakes*
- *2-3 green onions, chopped*

Directions

1. Heat oil in a large pot over medium-high.
2. Add garlic and yellow onion, and cook for 2-3 minutes, stirring.
3. Add broth, amino acids, and frozen wontons.
4. Bring to a boil, then reduce heat to medium.
5. Add rice noodles when wontons start to thaw.
6. Add shredded chicken and mix well.
7. Season with salt, pepper, and lime juice.
8. Let simmer for a couple minutes more, until the noodles are al dente.
9. Serve hot with green onion. Enjoy!

KALE MUSHROOM SOUP

SERVINGS: 6-8   PREP TIME: 5 min.   COOK TIME: 5 min.

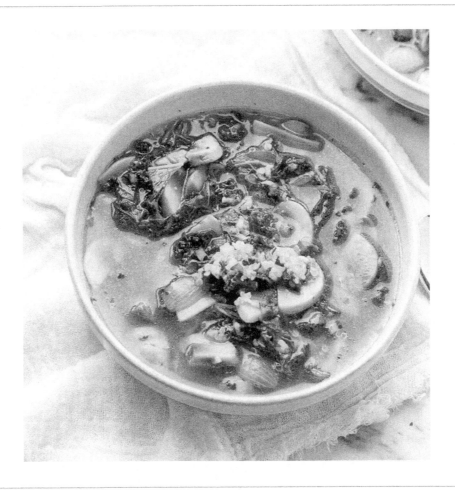

CARBS – 23 g   FAT – 3 g   PROTEIN – 6 g   CALORIES – 142

Ingredients

- 1 Tbsp coconut oil
- 1 large yellow onion, chopped
- 6 garlic cloves, minced
- 2 celery stalks, sliced
- 1 lb shitake mushrooms, chopped and stem bottoms removed
- ½ head kale, chopped
- ¼ tsp black pepper
- 1½ tsp sea salt
- 12 cups water
- 1 tsp turmeric
- 4 heads baby bok choy, bottoms cut off
- 1 Tbsp freshly grated ginger

Directions

1. Heat oil in a large pot over medium.
2. Add onions and cook for 5 minutes.
3. Add garlic and cook for 1 minute.
4. Add celery and mushrooms. Cook for 10 minutes.
5. Add spices, ginger, and water. Bring to boil.
6. Cover with lid and simmer for 50 minutes.
7. Add bok choy and kale, and cook 10 minutes more.
8. Serve warm.
9. Enjoy!

VEGETABLE RAMEN

SERVINGS: 6   PREP TIME: 15 min.   COOK TIME: 30 min.

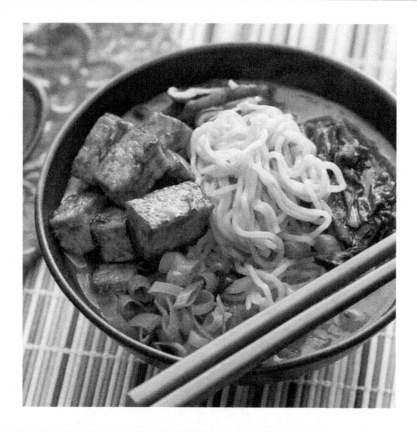

CARBS – 25 g   FAT – 10 g   PROTEIN – 19 g   CALORIES – 266

Ingredients

- *1 Tbsp toasted sesame oil*
- *6 cups water*
- *4 cups vegetable broth*
- *3 green onions, sliced*
- *3 oz shiitake mushrooms, thinly sliced*
- *1 4-inch turmeric root, peeled and grated*
- *5 cups shredded Napa cabbage*
- *1.5-inch ginger, peeled and grated*
- *7 oz enoki mushrooms, stems removed*
- *⅓ cup soy sauce*
- *3oz ramen noodles*

For the toppings:
- *2 tsp toasted sesame oil, divided*
- *6 baby bok choy, sliced in half*
- *1 lb tofu, diced*
- *2 tsp soy sauce*

Directions

1. Heat sesame oil in a pot.
2. Add green onions and shiitake mushrooms. Cook for 3 minutes.
3. Add cabbage. Cook for 4 minutes, stirring.
4. Add broth, water, ginger, turmeric, enoki mushrooms, and soy sauce. Bring to boil.
5. Add noodles and cover with the lid.
6. Simmer for 20 minutes on low heat.
7. Preheat 1 Tbsp sesame oil in a skillet.
8. Add bok choy (flat side down) and cook for 3-5 minutes over medium-high. Flip and cook 2 minutes more. Set aside.
9. Heat remaining oil and add tofu. Cook for 3-4 minutes, tossing.
10. Add soy sauce. Cook for 1 minute more
11. Serve soup with bok choy, tofu, and green onion on top.
12. Enjoy!

MUSTARD GLAZED SALMON AND ZOODLES

SERVINGS: 4   PREP TIME: 10 min.   COOK TIME: 10 min.

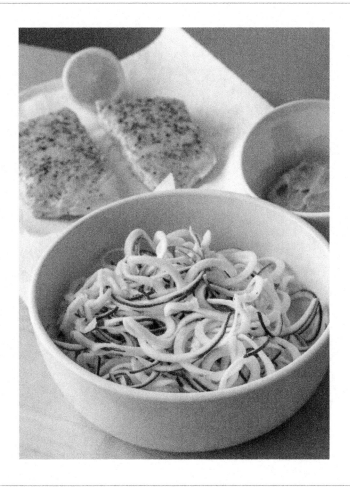

CARBS – 18 g   FAT – 10 g   PROTEIN – 30 g   CALORIES – 280

Ingredients

- *1 lb wild sockeye salmon, boneless*
- *¼ cup dijon mustard*
- *1 Tbsp honey*
- *1 Tbsp lemon juice*
- *8 cups zucchini noodles*
- *1 Tbsp olive oil*
- *1 tsp lemon juice*
- *1 Tbsp coconut aminos*

Directions

1. Preheat oven to 425°F.
2. Put salmon, skin side down, on a baking sheet with parchment paper.
3. Mix Dijon mustard, honey, and lemon juice in a bowl. Coat salmon with half of the sauce.
4. Bake until salmon is cooked (10 minute).
5. Add oil to a baking sheet and place zoodles on top.
6. Sprinkle them with aminos and lemon juice.
7. Bake for 5 minutes.
8. Serve with remaining Dijon mustard.
9. Enjoy!

MISO SOUP

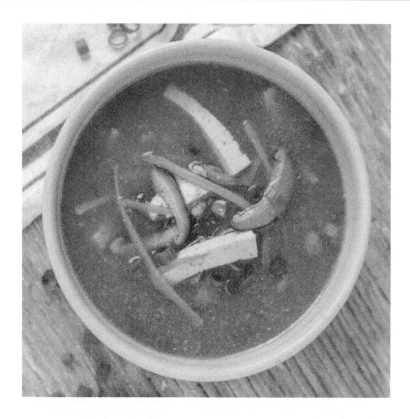

CARBS – 20 g   FAT – 1 g   PROTEIN – 2 g   CALORIES – 120

Ingredients

- 2 tbs olive oil
- 1 tbs fresh turmeric
- 3 tbs fresh ginger, grated
- 6 cloves garlic, minced
- 1 white onion, chopped
- 2 cups rainbow chard
- 3 tbs white miso paste
- ¼ cup fresh parsley, chopped
- 1 tsp salt, pepper
- 4 carrots, sliced into rounds
- 3 stalks celery, sliced thin
- 8 oz mushrooms, sliced
- 3 jalapenos, cut in half and sliced
- 2 lemons, juiced
- 1 tsp soy sauce
- 1 tbs apple cider vinegar
- 2 tbs ground turmeric
- 5 cups vegetable stock
- 1 (14 oz) block tofu, sliced into ½ inch squares

Directions

1. Heat oil in a large pot over medium.
2. Add onions, mushrooms, and celery. Cook for 8-9 minutes, stirring.
3. Add garlic, turmeric, and ginger. Cook for 5 minutes more.
4. In a bowl, mix miso paste, soy sauce, lemon juice, vinegar, salt, pepper, and ground turmeric. Adjust thickness with water.
5. Add carrot and tofu to the pot, and stir well.
6. Add the sauce and toss to coat vegetables.
7. After 3 minutes, pour in the stock and let it boil. Simmer for 20 minutes on low heat.
8. Pour in a bowl and serve hot.
9. Enjoy!

POTATOES AND GREEN BEANS WITH TUNA STEAK

SERVINGS: 2   PREP TIME: 25 min.   COOK TIME: 25 min.

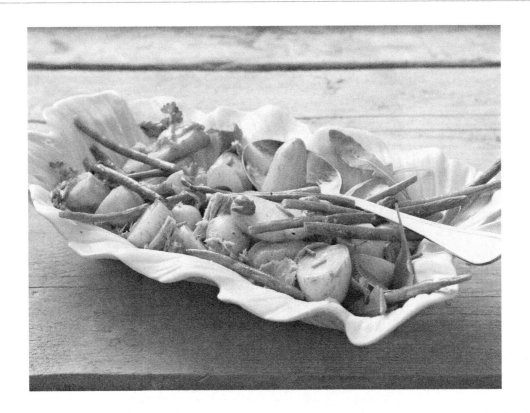

CARBS – 42 g   FAT – 4 g   PROTEIN – 9 g   CALORIES – 493

Ingredients

- *6 oz baby potatoes*
- *6 oz green beans*
- *¼ cup fresh lemon juice*
- *2½ Tbsp parsley minced*
- *1 Tbsp thyme*
- *2 Tbsp shallots, minced*
- *2 Tbsp unsalted chicken stock*
- *1½ tsp fresh rosemary minced*
- *4 tsp olive oil*
- *1 tsp Dijon mustard*
- *¼ tsp kosher salt*
- *¼ tsp black pepper*
- *8 oz tuna steak*

Directions

1. Cover potatoes with water in a pot. Bring to a boil over medium-high heat.
2. Boil the potatoes for 7 minutes.
3. Add green beans. Cook for 3 minutes.
4. Drain and rinse vegetables, and transfer to a bowl.
5. In another bowl, mix parsley, thyme, shallots, chicken stock, rosemary, olive oil, mustard, salt, and pepper. Stir well.
6. Cover the potatoes with half of herb mix.
7. Heat a cast-iron skillet over medium-high heat.
8. Season tuna steak with salt and pepper, coat with cooking spray.
9. Spray the skillet and add tuna.
10. Cook for 1 minute and 30 seconds each side for rare steak.
11. Serve potatoes and green beans with sliced tuna steak and remaining dressing. Enjoy!

GARLIC PASTA

SERVINGS: 4   PREP TIME: 15 min.   COOK TIME: 1 h. 45 min.

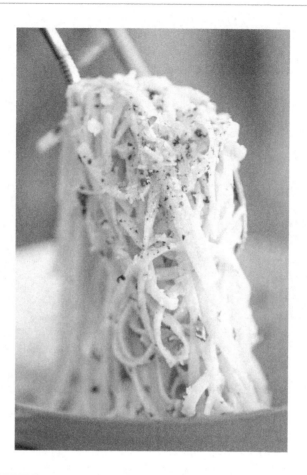

CARBS – 33 g   FAT – 32 g   PROTEIN – 11 g   CALORIES – 451

Ingredients

- *1 large head of garlic*
- *10 cloves, half sliced and half minced*
- *½ cup olive oil*
- *½ tsp dried red chili peppers*
- *¾ lb dried pasta*
- *5 cups low sodium chicken broth*
- *½ cup grated pecorino romano cheese*
- *2 Tbsp fresh lemon juice*
- *¼ cup freshly chopped parsley leaves*
- *Salt & cracked black pepper to taste*

Directions

1. Preheat oven to 350°F.
2. Cut off the top of the head of garlic and place it in a small oven-proof dish.
3. Coat with half of the olive oil, then cover with foil. Bake for 1 hour 30 minutes.
4. Heat remaining oil in a skillet over medium heat.
5. Add sliced garlic and cook until golden.
6. Remove from pan and set aside.
7. Add minced garlic and cook for 2 minutes.
8. Add chili peppers and broth. Bring to a boil.
9. Add pasta and cook until al dente.
10. Add cheese, sliced garlic, lemon juice, and parsley.
11. Squeeze the garlic head into the pan.
12. Add salt and pepper. Toss to coat pasta with sauce. Enjoy!

COCONUT CURRY SALMON

SERVINGS: 2   PREP TIME: 5 min.   COOK TIME: 5 min.

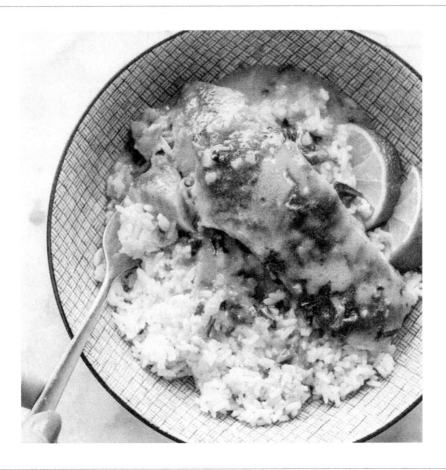

CARBS – 32 g   FAT – 15 g   PROTEIN – 32 g   CALORIES – 395

Ingredients

- 2 garlic cloves
- 6 scallions, white parts only
- 1 Tbsp curry powder
- 2 roasted red peppers
- Zest and juice of 2 limes
- 2-inch piece of ginger, peeled and chopped
- 2 Tbsp coconut vinegar
- 1 Tbsp soy sauce
- 2 Tbsp dark brown sugar
- 1 (15-ounce) can coconut milk
- 1 tsp kosher salt
- ½ tsp freshly ground black pepper
- ¼ cup cilantro leaves
- 1 lime, sliced thinly
- ⅓ cup toasted coconut
- 6 salmon fillets, deboned and skinned
- Kosher salt, to adjust in the end
- Freshly ground black pepper, to adjust in the end

Directions

1. Preheat oven to 300°F.
2. Lightly oil a large casserole dish.
3. Blend scallions, garlic, ginger, curry, red peppers, lime zest, juice, vinegar, soy sauce, sugar, milk, salt, and pepper in a blender to make a thick sauce.
4. Season fillets with salt and pepper, then place in the dish. Pour about 2/3 of sauce over fish.
5. Bake for 20 minutes, uncovered.
6. Serve hot with lime, cilantro, and remaining sauce.
7. Enjoy!

BUTTERNUT SQUASH KALE SOUP

SERVINGS: 4-6   PREP TIME: 5 min.   COOK TIME: 5 min.

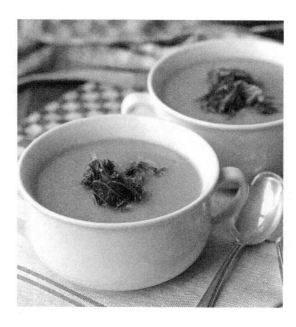

CARBS – 25 g   FAT – 3 g   PROTEIN – 17 g   CALORIES – 193

Ingredients

- *1 butternut squash, deseeded, peeled, and cut into bite-size cubes*
- *1 Tbsp melted coconut oil*
- *½ cup chickpeas, soaked overnight, drained*
- *4-inch piece kombu*
- *9 cups purified water*
- *2 lemongrass stalks, chopped*
- *3 garlic cloves, sliced*
- *1-inch piece fresh ginger, peeled and diced*
- *1 tsp ground turmeric*
- *1 small chili, seeded and minced*
- *½ bunch cilantro, stems and leaves separated*
- *2 lemons*
- *3 large kale leaves, stems removed and leaves chopped*
- *1 Tbsp tamari*

Directions

1. Preheat oven to 400°F.
2. Line a rimmed baking sheet with parchment paper.
3. Place squash on the baking sheet, and season with salt and pepper, drizzle with oil.
4. Bake for 20-30 minutes. Take out, set aside.
5. Add chickpeas, kombu, and water to the pot. Bring it to boil, skimming foam.
6. Cook for 30 minutes, simmering it.
7. Drain broth to pot and set aside chickpeas.
8. Add lemongrass, garlic, ginger, turmeric, chili to the broth. Let it boil.
9. Cover with lid and let simmer for 10 minutes.
10. Remove from heat, add lemon juice, and let it sit for 30 minutes, covered.
11. Strain the broth through a sieve into a heatproof bowl and discard the solids. Pour the broth back into the pot.
12. Add chickpeas and kale to the broth.
13. Bring it to boil and simmer for 5 minutes.
14. Add squash and let it heat through.
15. Add lemon juice and tamari.
16. Serve hot and enjoy!

SPRING VEGETABLE CHICKEN SOUP

SERVINGS: 2   PREP TIME: 10 min.   COOK TIME: 10 min.

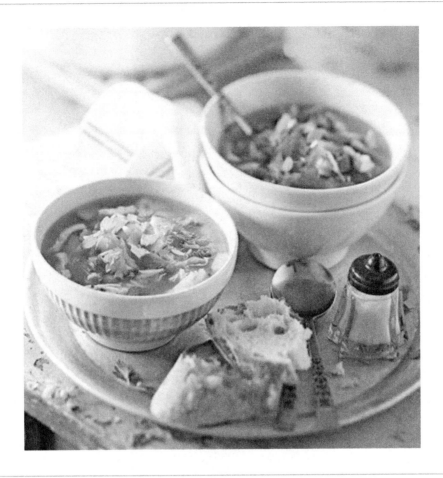

CARBS – 28 g   FAT – 17 g   PROTEIN – 43 g   CALORIES – 465

Ingredients

- 1 Tbsp olive oil
- 1 large chicken breast, skin on
- 500 ml chicken stock
- 1 slice sourdough bread, cut into cubes
- 2 Tbsp grated parmesan
- 2 large handfuls spring greens, finely sliced
- 4 asparagus spears, trimmed and halved
- 40 g peas
- 400 g can borlotti beans, drained and rinsed

Directions

1. Heat oven to 365°F.
2. Heat oil in a pan over medium.
3. Add chicken and brown on each side.
4. Remove chicken and pour in the stock.
5. Let it boil, then add back the chicken. Cook for 5 mins.
6. Cover with lid and let it sit for 30 minutes.
7. Spread bread cubes on a baking tray.
8. Drizzle with oil, salt, and parmesan.
9. Bake for 6 minutes until golden.
10. Take out chicken and slice it.
11. Bring stock to boil and add greens, peas, and asparagus. Cook for 1 minute.
12. Add beans and sliced chicken.
13. Heat the soup sond serve it with crunchy parmesan cubes. Enjoy!

BROCCOLI ASPARAGUS RICE

SERVINGS: 4   PREP TIME: 5 min.   COOK TIME: 5 min.

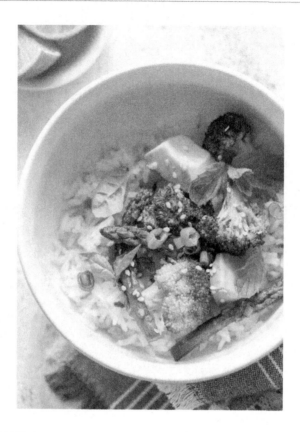

CARBS – 18 g   FAT – 4 g   PROTEIN – 6 g   CALORIES – 126

Ingredients

- *1 cup cooked jasmin rice*
- *1 cup broccoli florets, bite-sized pieces*
- *1 cup asparagus, bite-sized pieces*
- *1 cup kale leaves, chopped, stems removed*
- *2 green onions, sliced*
- *2 garlic cloves, chopped*
- *1 tsp fresh ginger, chopped*
- *½ Tbsp extra virgin olive oil*
- *¼ tsp toasted sesame oil*
- *½ tsp tamari, low sodium*
- *1 egg*
- *1 avocado, diced*

Directions

1. Heat the oil in a pan on medium-high.
2. Add garlic, green onion (white parts), and ginger. Cook for 1 minute, stirring.
3. Add asparagus, kale, and broccoli .
4. Cook for 5 minutes, until leaves starts to wilt.
5. Add rice and green onion (green parts). Cook for 2-3 minutes, stirring.
6. Push rice and veggies to one side of the pan and beat the egg on the clean side.
7. Scramble the egg and mix it with rice and veggies.
8. Reduce heat to low and add sesame oil and tamari. Stir for 1-2 minutes.
9. Serve hot with diced avocado. Enjoy!

SPROUTS

SERVINGS: 2   PREP TIME: 15 min.   COOK TIME: 15 min.

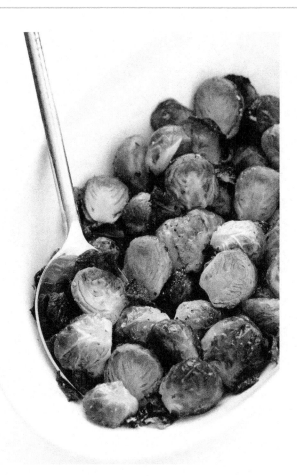

CARBS – 4 g   FAT – 18 g   PROTEIN – 12 g   CALORIES – 99

Ingredients

- *10 Brussel sprouts, halved*
- *2 bacon slices, chopped*
- *2 Tbsp butter*
- *Salt and pepper, to taste*

Directions

1. Steam sprouts for 10 minutes.
2. Heat a pan and melt butter over medium-high heat.
3. Cook bacon for 2 minutes, until crispy and brown.
4. Add sprouts. Cook for 3 minutes, stirring.
5. Season with salt and pepper. Mix well.
6. Remove from heat and serve.
7. Enjoy!

BUDDHA RICE BOWL WITH TAHINI DRESSING

SERVINGS: 4-6   PREP TIME: 10 min.   COOK TIME: 10 min.

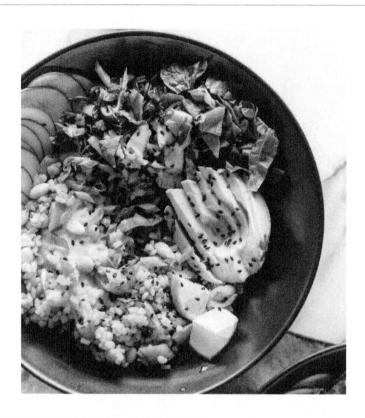

CARBS – 68 g   FAT – 31 g   PROTEIN – 34 g   CALORIES – 683

Ingredients

- 1 cup short-grain brown rice, cooked
- 2 cups water or vegetable stock
- 4 Tbsp extra-virgin olive oil
- Freshly ground pepper
- 2 cups peeled, cubed butternut
- 1 medium yellow onion, thinly sliced
- 6 cups kale, ribs discarded, leaves chopped
- ¼ cup tahini
- Juice of 1 lemon
- 1 tsp grated ginger
- 1½ tsp honey
- 1½ tsp sea salt
- ¾ cup hot water
- 1 pinch of sesame seeds, toasted
- 1 avocado, sliced

Directions

1. Preheat oven to 375°F.
2. Season squash with 2 Tbsp oil, salt, and pepper.
3. Place squash on a baking tray and bake for 20–25 minutes.
4. Heat 2 Tbsp oil in a large pan.
5. Add onions and brown them. Stir and lower the heat.
6. Caramelize onions for 15 minutes.
7. Remove onions and set aside.
8. Add kale to the pan and season with salt. Cook until it starts to soften.
9. Add tahini, lemon, ginger, honey, and ½ tsp salt. Stir.
10. Adjust the thickness of sauce with water if needed.
11. Serve with cooked brown rice, onions, squash, avocado slices, and kale.
12. Sprinkle with toasted sesame seeds. Enjoy!

TOMATO SAUCE WITH MUSHROOMS

SERVINGS: 1   PREP TIME: 20 min.   COOK TIME: 30 min.

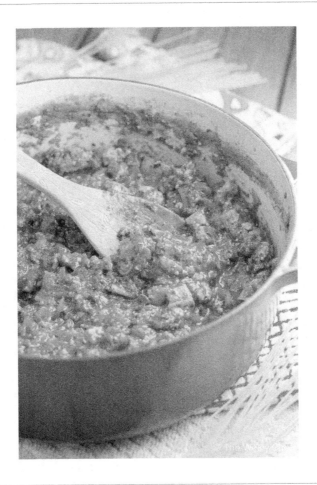

CARBS – 6 g   FAT – 1 g   PROTEIN – 1 g   CALORIES – 40

Ingredients

- 1 Tbsp extra-virgin olive oil
- 1 sweet onion, diced
- 4 cloves garlic, minced
- 8 ounces cremini mushrooms, sliced
- ½ cup packed fresh basil, chopped
- 1 can diced tomatoes + juices
- 6 Tbsp tomato paste
- 1 tsp sea salt
- 1½ tsp dried oregano
- ½ tsp dried thyme
- 2 Tbsp chia seeds

Directions

1. Heat oil in a saucepan over medium heat.
2. Add onion and garlic. Season with salt and pepper. Cook for 5-6 minutes.
3. Add mushrooms and increase heat to medium-high. Cook for 5-10 minutes, until liquid is cooked off.
4. Add basil, tomatoes, juice, tomato paste, salt, oregano, and thyme. Mix well.
5. Add chia seeds and stir.
6. Reduce heat and simmer for 15-20 minutes, stirring.
7. Serve with your favorite pasta or zoodles.
8. Enjoy!

PISTACHIO BUDDHA BOWL

SERVINGS: 2   PREP TIME: 10 min.   COOK TIME: 30 min.

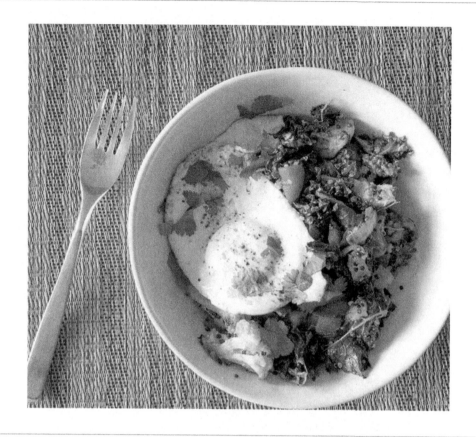

CARBS – 24 g   FAT – 17 g   PROTEIN – 19 g   CALORIES – 563

Ingredients

For Pistachio Spice Blend:
- ½ cup pistachios, finely chopped
- ¼ cup raw sesame seeds
- 1½ Tbsp coriander seeds
- 1 Tbsp cumin seeds
- 3 Tbsp hemp seeds
- ¼ tsp black pepper
- 1 tsp salt

For Buddha Bowl:
- ⅔ cup cooked any grain
- 2 handfuls microgreens
- 1 bunch seasonal fresh veggies of choice, sliced
- 2 Tbsp olive oil
- ½ lemon
- 1 soft-boiled egg
- 2 Tbsp favorite dressing (optional)

Directions

1. Heat a pan over medium-high heat.
2. Add sesame seeds and toast for 5 minutes.
3. Remove seeds to a bowl and add cumin and coriander to the pan. Cook for 1-2 minutes.
4. Grind cumin, coriander, and sesame seeds and mix together. Place them in the jar.
5. Add hemp seeds, pistachios, salt, and pepper to the jar. Shake well.
6. Divide cooked grain between 2 bowls.
7. Top with preferred veggies and drizzle with lemon juice and olive oil.
8. Serve with half of the egg, sprinkle with pistachio spice.
9. Enjoy!

SALADS AND SNACKS

FALL SALAD

SERVINGS: 6   PREP TIME: 10 min.   COOK TIME: 10 min.

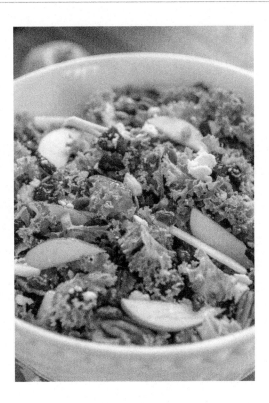

CARBS – 17 g   FAT – 7 g   PROTEIN – 4 g   CALORIES – 150

Ingredients

- *1 bunch kale, thinly sliced*
- *1 apple, sliced into matchsticks*
- *1 small pomegranate*

For the dressing:
- *3 Tbsp olive oil*
- *4 Tbsp apple cider vinegar*
- *Juice of 1 lemon*
- *1 Tbsp mustard*
- *1 Tbsp honey*

For pecans:
- *1 cup pecans, chopped*
- *1 Tbsp coconut oil*
- *½ Tbsp maple syrup*
- *¼ tsp salt*

Directions

1. Preheat oven to 375°F.
2. Line baking tray with parchment paper.
3. Mix 3 Tbsp vinegar, juice of half lemon, mustard, olive oil and honey in a large bowl.
4. Add kale to and toss to coat evenly.
5. Mix remaining lemon juice and vinegar in a bowl. Add apples and coat with mixture.
6. In another bowl mix ingredients for the pecans.
7. Spread pecans on baking tray and bake for 7-8 minutes. Take out and let them cool.
8. Combine all the prepared ingredients together to get fall salad.
9. Enjoy!

LEMON GINGER BITES

SERVINGS: 6   PREP TIME: 10 min.   COOK TIME: 10 min.

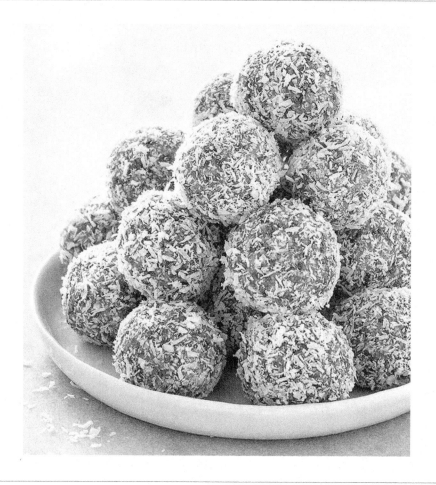

CARBS – 21 g   FAT – 6 g   PROTEIN – 2 g   CALORIES – 150

Ingredients

- *1 cup Medjool dates, pitted*
- *1 cup pecans*
- *½ cup hemp seeds, plus more for coating*
- *½ cup unsweetened coconut flakes, plus more for coating*
- *Zest and juice of 1 lemon*
- *1 Tbsp freshly grated ginger*
- *1 tsp vanilla extract*
- *Pinch of salt*

Directions

1. Chop pecans in a food processor.
2. Add all ingredients to the pecans and pulse until it starts to stick together.
3. Make small balls from the mixture.
4. Roll balls in coconut flakes or hemp seeds to coat them.
5. Transfer to an air-tight container and keep in the fridge for 1 week.
6. Enjoy!

ORANGE CHICKEN SALAD

SERVINGS: 2   PREP TIME: 10 min.   COOK TIME: 35 min.

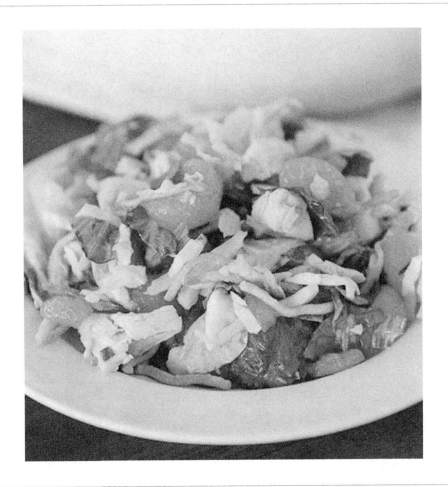

CARBS – 40 g   FAT – 8 g   PROTEIN – 21 g   CALORIES – 307

Ingredients

- ¾ cup light sesame ginger dressing
- 2 tsp toasted sesame oil, divided
- ¼ cup orange juice
- 3 cups chopped romaine lettuce
- 2 skinless and boneless chicken breasts
- ½ bag coleslaw mix
- ½ cup pistachios, crushed
- 2 mandarins wedges, for serving
- ¼ cup jicama, sliced

Directions

1. Combine ¼ cup dressing, 1 tsp sesame oil, and orange juice in ziplock bag.
2. Put the chicken in the bag and marinate overnight.
3. Oil a baking sheet using cooking spray.
4. Remove chicken from the marinade and put it on the baking sheet.
5. Bake chicken at for 30-35 minutes, until there is no longer pink meat. Cut the meat.
6. Combine pistachios, coleslaw mix, ¼ cup dressing jicama, 1 tsp sesame oil in a bowl.
7. Place slaw on the plate with chicken on top of it. Drizzle with ¼ cup dressing.
8. Enjoy!

KALE, BEET AND TUNA SALAD

SERVINGS: 1   PREP TIME: 5 min.   COOK TIME: 5 min.

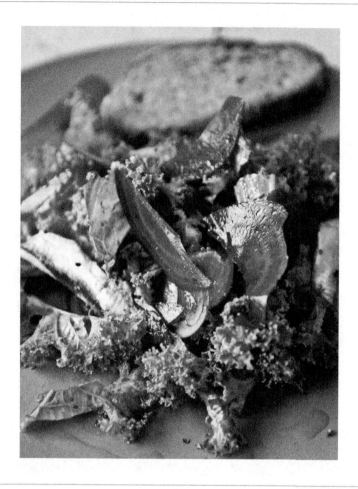

CARBS – 27 g   FAT – 15 g   PROTEIN – 21 g   CALORIES – 324

Ingredients

- *2 Tbsp fresh lemon juice*
- *2 Tbsp olive oil*
- *1 tsp drained capers*
- *½ tsp Dijon mustard*
- *3 cups baby kale*
- *½ roasted haricots verts, cut into 1-inch pieces*
- *½ roasted beet wedges*
- *⅛ tsp kosher salt*
- *1 pouch low-sodium tuna in water*

Directions

1. Combine oil, capers, lemon juice, and mustard in a large bowl.
2. Add haricot verts, kale, beets, salt to the bowl.
3. Toss well to coat the ingredients evenly.
4. Place tuna on top of the salad.
5. Serve immediately.
6. Enjoy!

HIJIKI AVOCADO SALAD

SERVINGS: 3   PREP TIME: 10 min.   COOK TIME: 10 min.

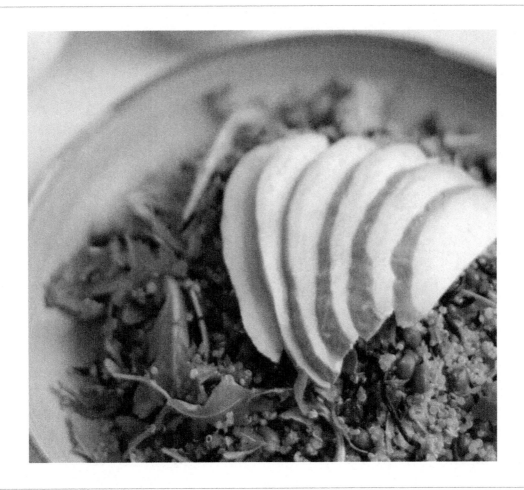

CARBS – 19 g   FAT – 10 g   PROTEIN – 3 g   CALORIES – 145

Ingredients

- *1 cup hijiki seaweed, drained (¼ cup + 1 Tbsp dried hijiki with ¾ cup water)*
- *2 cups cooked quinoa*
- *1 (15 oz) can adzuki beans, rinsed and drained*
- *1 ripe avocado, cut into cubes*

For the dressing:

- *2 Tbsp reduced-sodium tamari soy sauce*
- *¼ cup rice vinegar*
- *1 Tbsp toasted sesame oil*

Directions

1. Soak the hijiki in a bowl for 15 minutes to reconstitute them.
2. Drain excess liquid from hijiki.
3. Mix tamari soy sauce, vinegar, and sesame oil in a large bowl.
4. Add quinoa, hijiki, adzuki beans to the bowl. Toss well to coat.
5. Place sliced avocado on top and serve.
6. Enjoy!

THYME ROASTED ALMONDS

SERVINGS: 6-8   PREP TIME: 5 min.   COOK TIME: 15 min.

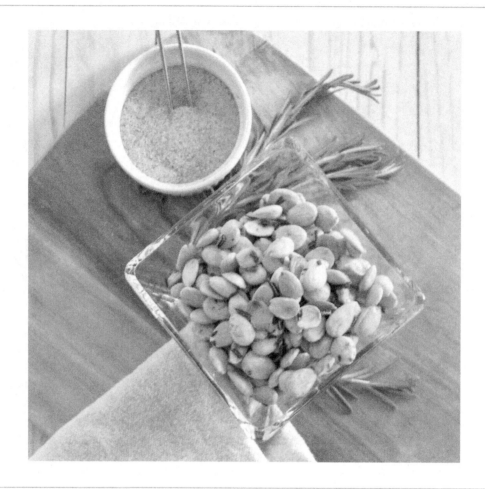

CARBS – 6 g   FAT – 15 g   PROTEIN – 6 g   CALORIES – 170

Ingredients

- *1 pound roasted, salted Marcona almonds*
- *2 tsp olive oil*
- *2 Tbsp thyme leaves, minced*
- *1 tsp fleur de sel*
- *1 tsp kosher salt*

Directions

1. Preheat the oven to 350°F.
2. Spread olive oil, almonds, thyme, and kosher salt on a sheet pan.
3. Toss everything together.
4. Roast for 10-15 minutes, stirring every 5 minutes with a spatula.
5. When done cooking, season with the fleur de sel and toss well.
6. Let the nuts cool.
7. Enjoy!

TUNA PITA POCKETS

SERVINGS: 4   PREP TIME: 15 min.   COOK TIME: 15 min.

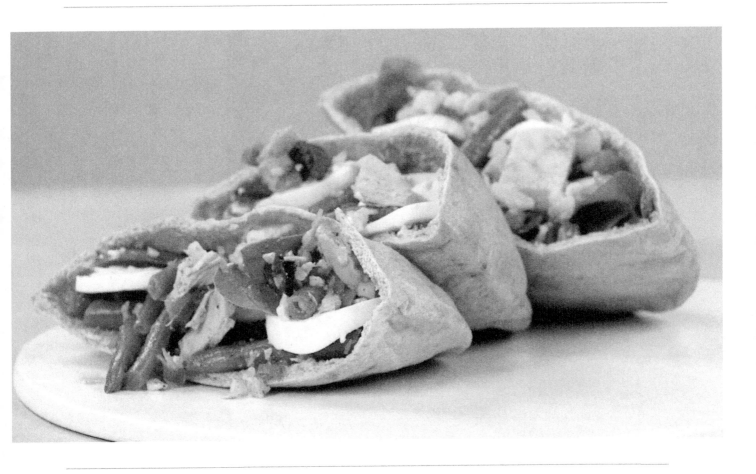

CARBS – 26 g   FAT – 14 g   PROTEIN – 18 g   CALORIES – 296

Ingredients

- 8 oz green beans, cooked and cut in half
- 2 cup chopped cauliflower, red peppers, onions (all together)
- 2 Tbsp olive oil
- 2 Tbsp fresh lemon juice
- ¼ tsp kosher salt
- ¼ tsp black pepper
- 1 can albacore tuna, broken into large flakes
- 6 pitted kalamata olives, sliced
- ¼ cup plain hummus
- 2 whole-wheat pitas, halved and toasted
- 1 cup baby spinach leaves
- 2 large hard-cooked eggs, sliced

Directions

1. Add green beans, peppers, onions, cauliflower, olive oil, juice, salt, black pepper, tuna, and olives in a bowl. Mix well to combine.
2. Spread 1-2 Tbsp hummus inside pitas.
3. Add ¼ cup spinach to each pita, then ½ tuna mixture.
4. Top with sliced egg.
5. Enjoy!

WATERMELON GREEN SALAD

SERVINGS: 4-6   PREP TIME: 30 min. + 2 weeks for tonic   COOK TIME: 30 min.

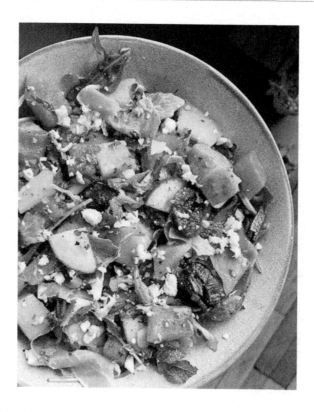

CARBS – 52 g   FAT – 8 g   PROTEIN – 4 g   CALORIES – 285

Ingredients

For the salad:
- *1 cup watermelon*
- *1 cup cucumber, sliced*
- *1 sliced avocado*
- *⅓ cup crumbled feta cheese*
- *1 cup baby broccoli*
- *½ cup toasted almonds*
- *4 cups baby kale or other greens*

For the immune-boosting tonic:
- *¼ cup garlic, minced*
- *¼ cup onion, chopped*
- *2 Tbsp horseradish, minced*
- *2 knobs turmeric, chopped*
- *1 jalapeno pepper, chopped*
- *32 oz organic apple cider vinegar*
- *¼ cup fresh ginger, chopped*
- *Juice of 1 lemon*

For the dressing:
- *½ cup olive oil*
- *½ cup master tonic*
- *¼ cup goji berries*
- *4 dates*

Directions

1. Combine all ingredients for the salad in a bowl and toss well.
2. To make tonic, combine all ingredients in a separate bowl. Mix well and transfer to a jar.
3. Let it sit for 1-2 weeks, shake occasionally.
4. Strain tonic and put the liquid back in the jar.
5. To make the dressing, combine the tonic, olive oil, and salt in a bowl.
6. Blend the goji berries and dates until smooth.
7. Drizzle salad with dressing and serve.

BERRY SPINACH SALAD

SERVINGS: 6   PREP TIME: 5 min.   COOK TIME: 5 min.

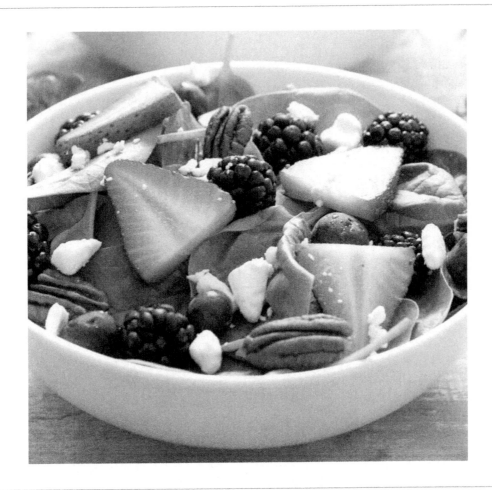

CARBS – 24 g   FAT – 31 g   PROTEIN – 6 g   CALORIES – 351

Ingredients

- 4 cups organic baby spinach
- 1 cup raspberries
- 1 cup blackberries
- 1 cup blueberries
- 1 cup almonds

For the dressing:
- ½ cup olive oil
- ¼ cup balsamic vinegar
- 1 tsp honey
- 1 tsp mustard
- 1 clove garlic, minced
- Salt and ground black pepper, to taste

Directions

1. Combine olive oil, vinegar, mustard, garlic, honey, salt, and black pepper in a bowl.
2. In another bowl, toss together spinach, berries, and almonds.
3. Drizzle salad lightly with dressing.
4. Enjoy!

VITAMIN C BITES

SERVINGS: 2   PREP TIME: 10 min.   COOK TIME: 35 min.

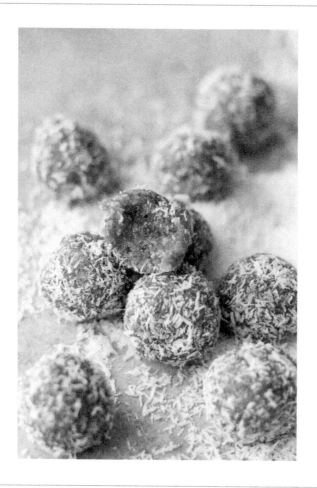

CARBS – 4 g   FAT – 21 g   PROTEIN – 11 g   CALORIES – 185

Ingredients

- *½ cup cashews*
- *½ cup almonds*
- *15 dates*
- *Coconut flakes*
- *3 sachets of organic vitamin c powder*

Directions

1. Add nuts and dates to a food processor and pulse until the start coming together.
2. Add powder to the mixture.
3. Make 10 balls.
4. Roll them in the coconut flakes.
5. Lay balls on a tray and refrigerate for 3 hours.
6. Enjoy!

WINTER CITRUS SALAD

SERVINGS: 6   PREP TIME: 10 min.   COOK TIME: 35 min.

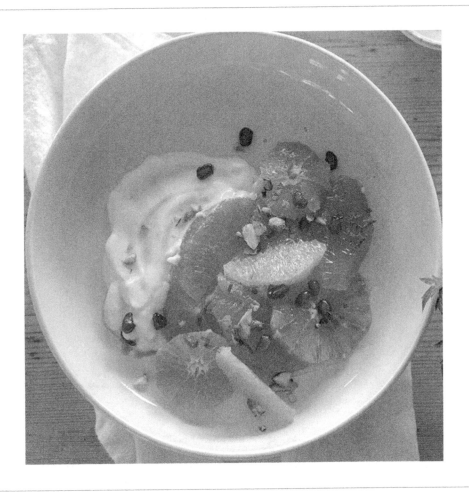

CARBS – 12 g   FAT – 0 g   PROTEIN – 1 g   CALORIES – 50

Ingredients

- 1 grapefruit, peeled and cut into wheels
- 1 navel orange, peeled and cut into wheels
- 1 Tbsp olive oil
- 1 tsp raw honey
- 4-5 fresh mint leaves, minced
- 2 Tbsp raw cashew pieces
- Pomegranate seeds for serving (optional)

Directions

1. Mix olive oil and honey in a bowl.
2. Add mint leaves to the honey mixture and let it sit for 10-15 minutes.
3. Combine citruses and cashew in another bowl.
4. Drizzle citrus salad lightly.
5. Serve with plain greek yogurt.
6. Enjoy!

CAJUN SALMON AND KALE SALAD

SERVINGS: 2   PREP TIME: 20 min.   COOK TIME: 20 min.

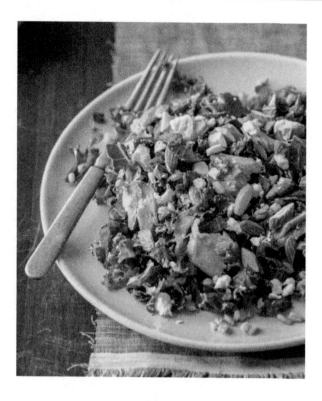

CARBS – 29 g   FAT – 35 g   PROTEIN – 38 g   CALORIES – 561

Ingredients

- *2 medium salmon fillets, skin on*
- *Coconut oil*

For the spice blend:
- *1 tsp paprika powder*
- *1 tsp coriander seed powder*
- *½ tsp cumin powder*
- *1 tsp onion powder*
- *½ tsp garlic powder*
- *1 tsp dried oregano*

For the salad:
- *5-6 oz shredded kale, stems removed and leaves sliced*
- *1 large carrot, grated*
- *½ red pepper, sliced*
- *1 green spring onion, chopped*
- *¼ cup pumpkin seeds*
- *¼ cup dried cranberries*
- *A handful of fresh parsley*

For the dressing:
- *Juice of ½ lime*
- *2 Tbsp olive oil*
- *1 tsp honey*
- *1 tsp dijon mustard*
- *A little salt and pepper*

Directions

1. Mix all the spice ingredients and rub onto salmon fillets.
2. Add dressing ingredients and kale leaves to a bowl and toss well.
3. Heat oil in a pan over medium-high heat.
4. Add fillets, skin side down. Cook for 5 minutes.
5. Flip fillets and cook for 2 minutes.
6. Add the rest of salad ingredients to kale leaves and mix well.
7. Cut salmon into bite size pieces and add to the salad.
8. Enjoy!

SALMON AVOCADO TOAST

SERVINGS: 2   PREP TIME: 5 min.   COOK TIME: 5 min.

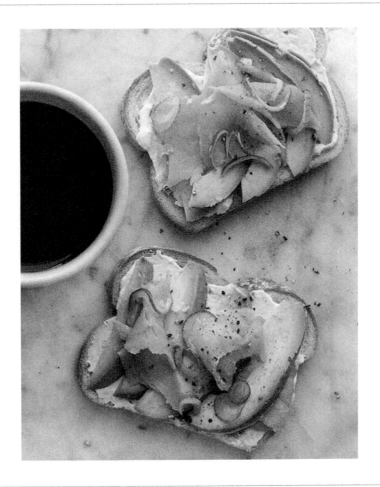

CARBS – 20 g   FAT – 17 g   PROTEIN – 11 g   CALORIES – 262

Ingredients

- 2 slices rustic bread, toasted
- 3 tsp less fat-free cream cheese
- ½ avocado, sliced
- 2 oz lox styled salmon
- 8 pieces red onion, thinly sliced
- Pinch of black pepper
- ¼ tsp capers

Directions

1. Spread toast with cream cheese.
2. Put avocado slices on top, then salmon slices, onion, and cappers.
3. Sprinkle with black pepper.
4. Enjoy!

SAUERKRAUT

SERVINGS: 1   PREP TIME: 5 min.   COOK TIME: 5 min.

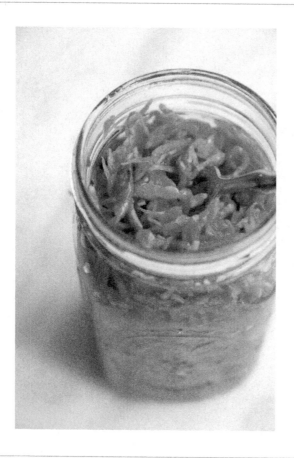

CARBS – 27 g   FAT – 7 g   PROTEIN – 26 g   CALORIES – 273

Ingredients

- *2 medium red or green cabbages, cores removed and thinly sliced*
- *3 Tbsp unrefined sea salt*

Directions

1. Sterilize a mason jar and lid by submerging it in boiling water for 10 minutes. Take out and drain it. Set aside.
2. Add cabbage to a large bowl and season with salt.
3. Squeeze cabbage with hands for 15 minutes to draw out the natural water .
4. Transfer cabbage and liquid to the jar.
5. If it's not enough liquid, add water. It should cover the cabbage.
6. When cabbage is submerged, lock the lid and leave it in a dark corner at room temperature for 1-3 weeks.
7. Cabbage is ready when it's soft and tastes tangy and sour.
8. Remove any white scum from the surface. Enjoy!

MUNG DAL

SERVINGS: 6   PREP TIME: 20 min.   COOK TIME: 40 min.

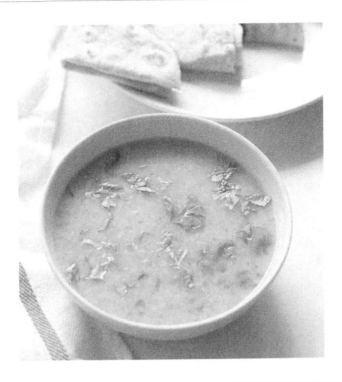

CARBS – 59 g   FAT – 1 g   PROTEIN – 25 g   CALORIES – 347

Ingredients

- 6 cups vegetable stock
- 18 oz green mung beans, soaked
- 1 Tbsp ground cumin
- 1 Tbsp ground turmeric
- 2 tsp ground coriander
- 6 cardamom pods, crushed
- 1 Tbsp ghee
- 4 onions, sliced
- 6 garlic cloves, grated
- 2 thumb-sized pieces ginger, grated
- 4 carrots, diced
- 2 celery sticks, diced
- 2 pinches sea salt
- 2 pinches black pepper
- 3 handfuls fresh cilantro, chopped
- 8 handfuls kale, stalks removed and sliced
- Juice of 1 lime or lemon

Directions

1. Bring stock to a boil in a large saucepan with a lid. Add the mung beans, and simmer over medium heat, covered, for 20 minutes.
2. Heat a pan and fry dry spices for 1 minute over medium-high heat, stirring.
3. Add ghee and onion. Cook for 10 minutes.
4. Add garlic and ginger. Fry for 5 minutes more.
5. After 20 minutes of mung beans boiling, add carrot, celery, onion, garlic, ginger mix.
6. Add salt, pepper, and chopped cilantro.
7. Cover with lid. Cook for 15 minutes over medium heat (add some water if needed)
8. Add sliced kale leaves and cook for a 2-3 minutes.
9. Serve hot with chopped cilantro. Enjoy!

EASTERN TUNA STEAK

SERVINGS: 2   PREP TIME: 5 min.   COOK TIME: 15 min.

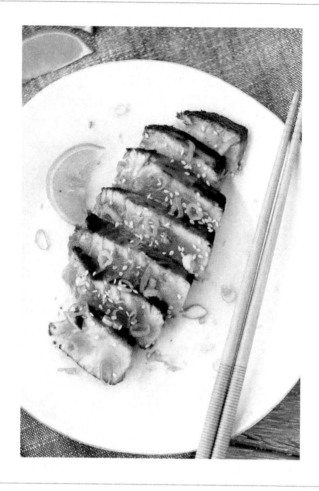

CARBS – 1 g   FAT – 18 g   PROTEIN – 34 g   CALORIES – 301

Ingredients

- *2 (5 oz) Ahi tuna steaks*
- *1½ Tbsp paprika*
- *½ Tbsp cayenne pepper*
- *¼ Tbsp freshly ground white pepper*
- *1 tsp whole peppercorns*
- *½ Tbsp butter*
- *2 Tbsp olive oil*
- *1 pinch chopped green onion*
- *1 tsp sesame seeds, toasted*

Directions

1. Mix paprika, cayenne, and white pepper in a bowl. Season steak on each side with mixture.
2. Heat oil with melted butter in a skillet over medium-high heat.
3. Add peppercorns and cook for 5 minutes.
4. Place tuna steak in the center of the skillet and cook for 1 minute each side (rare).
5. Slice tuna steak and serve with chopped green onion and sesame seeds.
6. Enjoy!

LEMON GINGER STIR-FRY

SERVINGS: 2   PREP TIME: 10 min.   COOK TIME: 20 min.

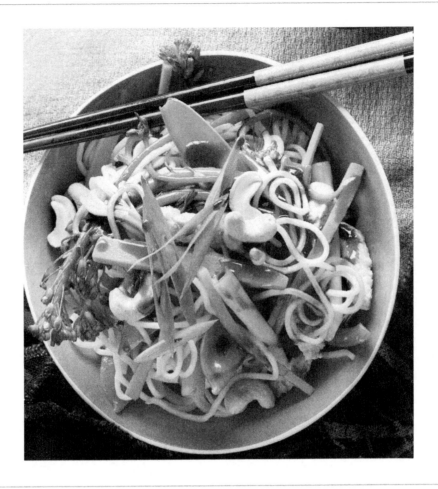

CARBS – 17 g   FAT – 5 g   PROTEIN – 5 g   CALORIES – 132

Ingredients

- *1 onion, diced*
- *1 garlic clove, crushed*
- *1 tsp sesame oil*
- *1 red bell pepper, cut into strips*
- *1 cup of boy choy, roughly chopped*
- *Juice and zest of 1 lemon*
- *1 Tbsp fresh ginger*
- *3 Tbsp honey*
- *3 Tbsp tamari*
- *2 Tbsp water*
- *2 Tbsp cashews*
- *1 package (2.6 oz) egg noodles, cooked*

Directions

1. Preheat the oil in a wok over medium-high heat.
2. Add garlic, onion, and all vegetables. Stir-fry for 2-3 minutes.
3. Add lemon juice, lemon zest, ginger, honey, tamari, and 1 Tbsp of water. Cook for 2 minutes.
4. Add cashews and noodles. Mix well.
5. Serve hot.
6. Enjoy!

TANDOORI SALMON WITH TOASTED GREENS

SERVINGS: 4   PREP TIME: 10 min.   COOK TIME: 15 min.

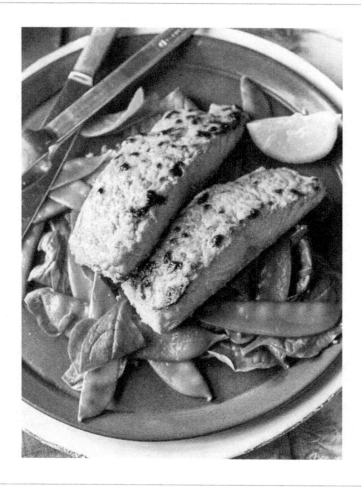

CARBS – 37 g   FAT – 26 g   PROTEIN – 35 g   CALORIES – 539

Ingredients

- 4 fillets skinless salmon fillets, bones removed
- 40 g gluten-free tandoori paste
- 1 cup green beans, halved
- 1½ cup mangetout
- 1½ cup baby spinach
- 1 Tbsp shredded or desiccated coconut, toasted
- 1 long red chili, finely sliced
- 2 Tbsp chopped coriander leaves
- 1 cup low-fat plain yogurt
- 1 garlic clove, crushed
- 1 tsp chopped dill

Directions

1. Coat salmon with tandoori paste.
2. Oil a non-stick pan with cooking spray and heat over medium heat.
3. Add salmon. Cook for 4 minutes each side.
4. Put salmon on a plate and let it rest for 5 minutes.
5. Wipe the pan, spray again, and heat.
6. Add beans and mangetout. Cook for 3 minutes.
7. Add spinach and cook until it wilts.
8. Add coconut and coriander. Season with pepper and mix well to combine.
9. Mix garlic, yogurt and dill in a bowl.
10. Serve salmon with herbed yogurt and lemon wedges. Enjoy!

TUNA POTATO PLATE

SERVINGS: 2   PREP TIME: 30 min.   COOK TIME: 45 min.

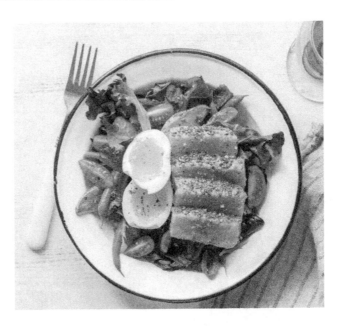

CARBS – 51 g   FAT – 24 g   PROTEIN – 29 g   CALORIES – 521

Ingredients

- 4 large eggs
- ½ lb small red potatoes
- ½ lb green beans
- 1 (8-oz) tuna steak
- ½ tsp kosher salt
- 1 cup rye berries
- ¾ tsp black pepper, divided
- ¼ cup + ½ tsp. extra-virgin olive oil
- 3 Tbsp fresh lemon juice
- 2 Tbsp shallot, minced
- 1 Tbsp fresh thyme, chopped
- 1½ tsp Dijon mustard
- ¼ cup flat-leaf parsley leaves
- 1 cup halved grape tomatoes, quartered

Directions

1. Place rye berries in a medium saucepan.
2. Add water to cover them by 1 inch.
3. Let it boil and cover with the lid.
4. Simmer for 5 minutes. Add eggs carefully.
5. Let it simmer for 7 minutes, covered.
6. Take out eggs with a slotted spoon and place in a bowl of ice water.
7. Cover the saucepan and cook for 20 minutes, stirring. Drain and rinse berries.
8. Peel eggs, and cut in half.
9. Put potatoes in a saucepan. Cover with 2 inches of water. Bring to boil.
10. Simmer for 10 minutes. Add green beans.
11. Simmer for 6 minutes , then take out the green beans and put in a bowl of ice water.
12. Cook potatoes for 3 minutes more.
13. Drain and rinse. Cut them into quarters.
14. Heat a cast-iron pan on medium-high heat.
15. Season tuna with salt and pepper, coat with cooking spray. Spray the skillet, add tuna.
16. Cook for 1 minute and 30 seconds each side for a rare steak. Slice steak thinly.
17. Whisk in a bowl oil, lemon juice, shallot, thyme, Dijon, and ¼ tsp pepper.
18. Mix rye berries, parsley, and half of dressing.
19. Top with green beans, potatoes, and tomatoes. Put tuna slices and egg halves on top of salad.
20. Drizzle with dressing. Enjoy!

CAULIFLOWER RICE

SERVINGS: 1   PREP TIME: 10 min.   COOK TIME: 10 min.

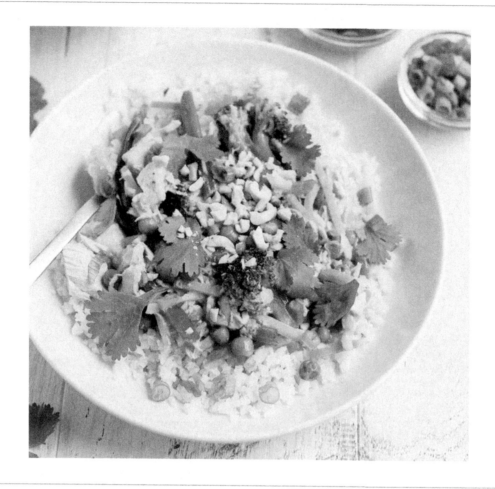

CARBS – 45 g   FAT – 5 g   PROTEIN – 16 g   CALORIES – 239

Ingredients

- 1 Tbsp coconut oil
- 1 medium cloves garlic, chopped
- 2 tsp grated fresh ginger
- ¼ cauliflower, cut into florets
- 1 cup capsicum, diced
- 2 spring onions, chopped
- 2 Tbsp fresh coriander, chopped
- 2 Tbsp desiccated coconut
- 1 Tbsp lemon juice
- 1 Tbsp soy sauce

Directions

1. Add florets to a food processor and pulse to get a fine crumble rice.
2. Heat oil in a large pan.
3. Add capsicum, cauliflower, garlic, ginger, and spring onions. Cook for about 1 minute.
4. Stir in coconut and lemon juice. Heat through.
5. Add soy sauce and stir well.
6. Serve hot with coriander leaves.
7. Enjoy!

TUNA WITH SALSA

SERVINGS: 2   PREP TIME: 5 min.   COOK TIME: 15 min.

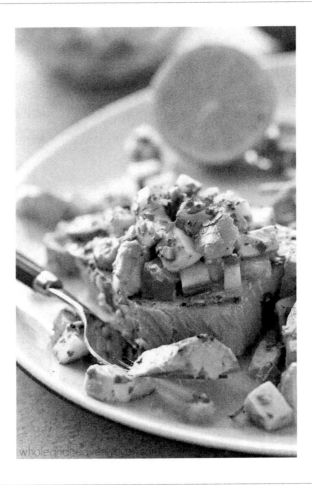

CARBS – 2 g   FAT – 3 g   PROTEIN – 18 g   CALORIES – 121

Ingredients

- *1 tuna fillet*
- *1 tomato, chopped*
- *Salt and pepper, to taste*
- *½ red onion finely, chopped*
- *1 Tbsp lime juice*
- *1 lemon juice*
- *1 avocado, cut into cubes*
- *½ red chili finely, chopped*
- *2 Tbsp olive oil*

Directions

1. Sprinkle fillet with salt and pepper, then coat with 1 Tbsp olive oil and lemon juice.
2. Mix onion, tomato, chili, avocado, lime juice, and 1 Tbsp olive oil in a bowl. Set aside.
3. Heat a frying pan over high heat.
4. Add tuna and cook for 3 minutes each side or more depending on thickness.
5. Serve tuna with salsa.
6. Enjoy!

GRILLED SPICED CHICKEN

SERVINGS: 2   PREP TIME: 5 min.   COOK TIME: 5 min.

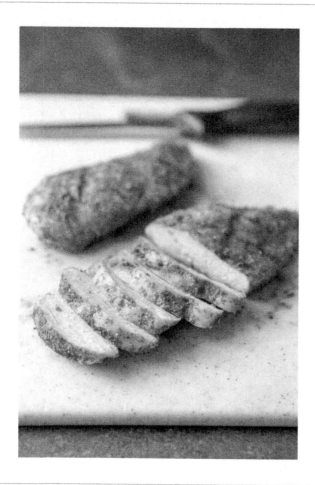

CARBS – 2 g   FAT – 8 g   PROTEIN – 22 g   CALORIES – 173

Ingredients

For the spice mix:
- *3 Tbsp turmeric*
- *1½ Tbsp ground cumin*
- *1½ Tbsp ground coriander*
- *1½ Tbsp ground fennel*
- *1½ tsp dry ginger*
- *1 tsp black pepper*
- *⅛ tsp cinnamon*
- *1½ tsp Celtic sea salt*

For the chicken:
- *2 chicken breasts*
- *3 Tbsp coconut oil, melted and divided*
- *1 Tbsp spice mix*

Directions

1. Combine all spice mix ingredients in a jar and shake well.
2. Heat a grill on high.
3. Rub chicken with coconut oil, then season each side with spice mix.
4. Oil the grill and add chicken.
5. Cook for 3 minutes until it's lightly browned.
6. Flip the chicken and fry for 3 minutes more.
7. Enjoy!

ROASTED CHICKEN SOUP

SERVINGS: 4   PREP TIME: 15 min.   COOK TIME: 1 h. 15 min.

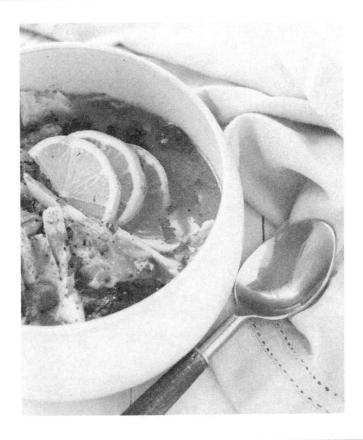

CARBS – 4 g   FAT – 0 g   PROTEIN – 8 g   CALORIES – 40

Ingredients

- 4 lb chicken, rinsed and dried
- 2 tsp salt
- 2 lemongrass stalks, ends trimmed, chopped
- ½ inch fresh ginger, sliced
- ½ inch fresh turmeric, sliced
- 9 cloves garlic
- 2 cups chicken broth
- 1 Tbsp unsalted butter
- 6 cups vegetables of choice chopped
- 1 handful parsley , chopped
- Lemon slices
- ¼ tsp ground turmeric

Directions

1. Preheat oven to 350°F.
2. Place chicken in a cast-iron dish with lid.
3. Add lemongrass, ginger, turmeric, and garlic to a mortar, and slightly crush.
4. Put some lemongrass mix to the bird cavity and place the rest around the chicken.
5. Pour broth over the chicken, then add butter and pepper.
6. Cover with foil and lid. Bake for 50 minutes.
7. Remove lid and foil, then spread vegetables around bird.
8. Cover with foil and lid. Bake for 30 minutes.
9. Remove from oven and let sit for 15 minutes.
10. Remove bird from the soup. Let it cool.
11. Shred the chicken and add it back to the soup.
12. Adjust salt and pepper, to taste.
13. Squeeze lemon juice and sprinkle with turmeric. Serve hot. Enjoy!

IMMUNE-BOOSTING GUMMIES

SERVINGS: 2   PREP TIME: 5 min.   COOK TIME: 5 min. + 2 h.

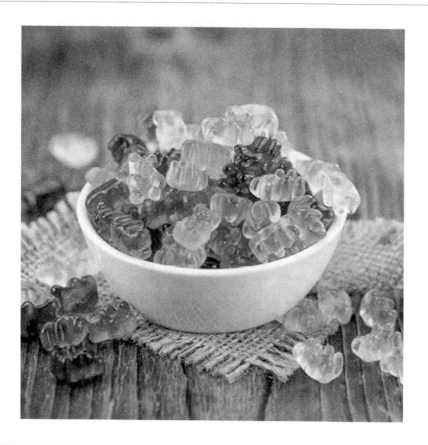

CARBS – 3 g   FAT – 0 g   PROTEIN – 0 g   CALORIES – 15

Ingredients

- *1½ cup organic apple juice*
- *1½ Tbsp raw honey*
- *3 Tbsp lemon juice*
- *6 scoops Flora's Elderberry Powder*
- *3 scoops Flora's Acerola Powder*
- *2 Tbsp gelatin*

Directions

1. Prepare silicone molds for gummies.
2. Pour apple juice into small saucepan on medium heat.
3. When it starts to steam, add lemon juice and honey. Mix well.
4. Turn off heat. Add elderberry and acerola powders, stirring until combined.
5. Add gelatin and whisk to dissolve it completely.
6. Pour mixture into the mold and refrigerate for 2-3 hours.
7. Remove gummies from mold and transfer to a mason jar.
8. Keep for a week in the fridge. Enjoy!

PUMPKIN SEED BARS

SERVINGS: 16   PREP TIME: 10 min.   COOK TIME: 15 min.

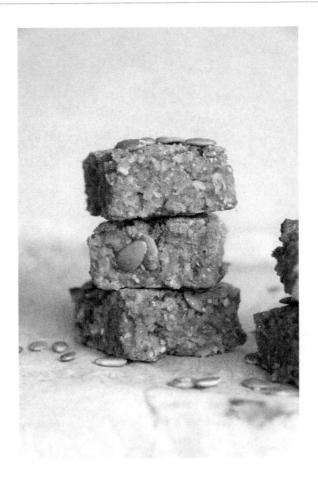

CARBS – 12 g   FAT – 12 g   PROTEIN – 8 g   CALORIES – 180

Ingredients

- 1 can (15 oz) chickpeas, drained and rinsed
- ½ cup dates
- ½ cup whole almonds
- 1 cup rolled oats
- ½ cup pumpkin puree
- ¼ cup maple syrup
- 2 Tbsp coconut oil
- ½ tsp baking soda
- 2 tsp baking powder
- 2 tsp vanilla
- 1½ tsp cinnamon
- ¼ cup rolled oats
- ¼ cup pumpkin seeds

Directions

1. Preheat the oven to 350°F.
2. Line a baking pan with parchment paper.
3. Add all ingredients except pumpkin seeds to a food processor and pulse to combine until smooth.
4. Spread mixture in one layer in pan.
5. Top with pumpkin seeds.
6. Bake for 15 minutes.
7. Store in the fridge for 2-3 days.
8. Enjoy!

FRUIT CUSTARD

SERVINGS: 6   PREP TIME: 15 min.   COOK TIME: 45 min.

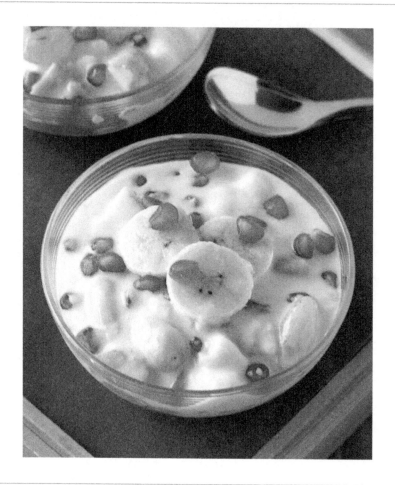

CARBS – 19 g   FAT – 0 g   PROTEIN – 5 g   CALORIES – 83

Ingredients

- 4 egg yolks
- 3 Tbsp sugar
- 400 ml milk
- 100 ml cream
- ½ tsp vanilla essence
- 4 green cardamom cloves
- 1 Tbsp flour, to thicken
- 1½ cups freshly cut fruit

Directions

1. Whisk egg yolks and sugar on a double boiler.
2. Add milk, cream, vanilla essence, and green cardamom in another pan. Mix well and let it sit for 5 minutes.
3. Add egg and sugar mixture to the pan. Cook on a slow heat and stir slowly, until it is thickened and there isn't any lumps form.
4. Mix flour and 2 Tbsp infused milk in a small bowl. Add it into the pan.
5. Strain custard to remove cardamom.
6. Put your preferred fruit in a bowl and pour over the custard.
7. Let it chill to smooth. Enjoy!

TURMERIC CHIA PUDDING

SERVINGS: 4   PREP TIME: 3 min.   COOK TIME: 4 h.

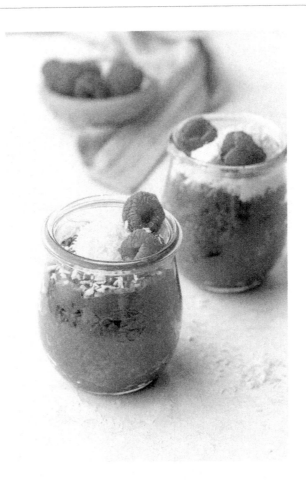

CARBS – 12 g   FAT – 10 g   PROTEIN – 5 g   CALORIES – 113

Ingredients

- ⅓ cup chia seeds
- 1 can full-fat coconut milk
- ¼ cup unsweetened cacao
- ½ tsp cinnamon
- 1 tsp ground turmeric
- 1-2 Tbsp raw honey
- ½ tsp vanilla extract

Directions

1. Put chia seeds, cacao powder, coconut milk, turmeric, cinnamon, vanilla, and raw honey in a blender and blend until smooth.
2. Cover and refrigerate for 4-5 hours to thicken.
3. Divide between 2 glasses and top with preferred toppings like fresh berries or coconut flakes.
4. Enjoy!

CITRUS CHIA PUDDING

SERVINGS: 1   PREP TIME: 5 min.   COOK TIME: 15 min.

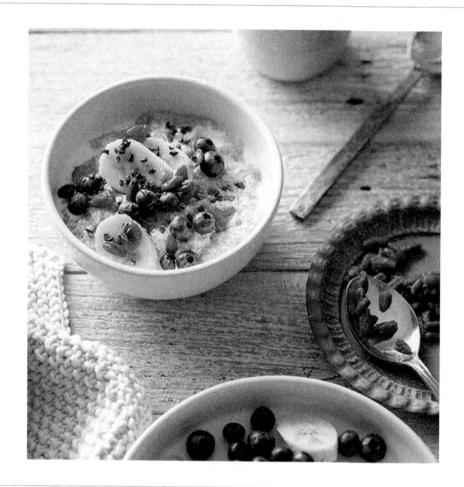

CARBS – 32 g   FAT – 9 g   PROTEIN – 6 g   CALORIES – 141

Ingredients

- *2 cups almond milk*
- *1 Tbsp ginger, grated*
- *Zest of 1 orange*
- *¼ cup fresh orange*
- *2 Tbsp maple syrup*
- *6 Tbsp chia seeds*
- *1 banana, sliced*
- *¼ cup blueberries*
- *¼ cup goji berries*

Directions

1. Put the almond milk, ginger, orange zest and juice, and maple syrup in a blender.
2. Blend until smooth.
3. Put chia seeds in a bowl and pour the blended mixture over them.
4. Give it a stir every 5 minutes during the next 20 minutes.
5. Refrigerate for 5-6 hours.
6. Top with banana slices and berries.
7. Enjoy!

APPLE TART

SERVINGS: 2   PREP TIME: 30 min.   COOK TIME: 10 min.

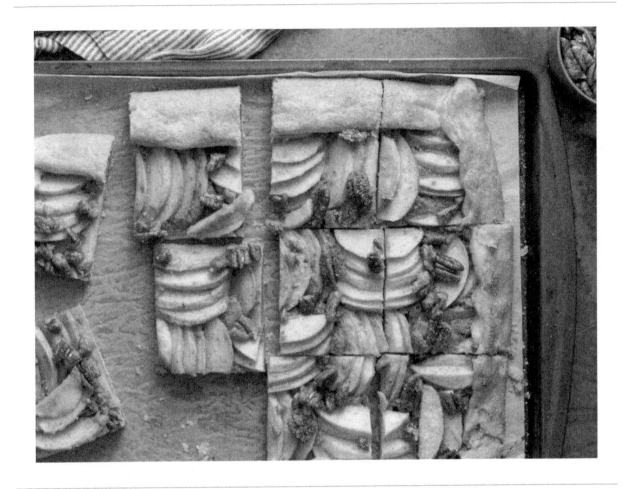

CARBS – 19 g   FAT – 8 g   PROTEIN – 3 g   CALORIES – 145

Ingredients

- 1 whole sheet puffed pastry, cut in half
- 1 cup brown sugar
- ¼ tsp salt
- Juice of ½ a lemon
- 3 whole apples, cored, halved and sliced
- ¼ cup pecans, sliced

Directions

1. Preheat oven to 425°F.
2. Line a baking sheet with parchment paper.
3. Spread puffed pastry rectangles on the prepared pan.
4. Mix apples, sugar, salt and lemon juice in a bowl. Let it sit for 5 minutes.
5. Arrange apple slices on the pastry in a line, overlapping
6. Bake for 20 minutes to make pastry golden brown.
7. Take out from the oven and serve hot.
8. Top with sliced pecans.
9. Enjoy!

BAKED APPLES

SERVINGS: 6   PREP TIME: 25 min.   COOK TIME: 1 h. 10 min.

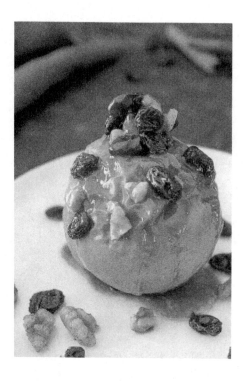

CARBS – 4 g   FAT – 15 g   PROTEIN – 3 g   CALORIES – 391

Ingredients

- *6 medium Golden Delicious apples*
- *1 cup walnut pieces*
- *½ cup raisins or dried cranberries*
- *2 Tbsp maple syrup*
- *1 tsp lemon zest*
- *¼ tsp ground cinnamon*
- *¼ tsp ground nutmeg*
- *½ cup apricot preserves*
- *1½ cup apple cider*
- *1 Tbsp butter*
- *½ tsp vanilla extract*

Directions

1. Preheat oven to 375° F.
2. Oil a baking dish with cooking spray.
3. Make a 1-inch-wide hole in each apple with an apple corer.
4. Using a sharp knife, make a crater from the hole on top of apples . Set apples aside.
5. Put walnuts and raisins in a food processor. Chop, but not too fine.
6. Add syrup, lemon zest, cinnamon,and nutmeg. Pulse a little to combine.
7. Put apples in the prepared baking dish.
8. Fill each cavity with enough filling.
9. Spoon preserves onto the crater of each apple.
10. Mix butter and cider in a small saucepan over low heat.
11. Remove from flame and add vanilla.
12. Pour the mixture over the apples and around them.
13. Cover apples with foil and bake for 30 minutes.
14. Take out and remove foil.
15. Baste apples and bake for 20-35 minutes more (depending on size).
16. Check apples for doneness – if you feel a little bit of resistance in the center with a bamboo skewer, they're done.
17. Enjoy!

GOJI BERRY BOWL

SERVINGS: 2   PREP TIME: 5 min.   COOK TIME: 5 min.

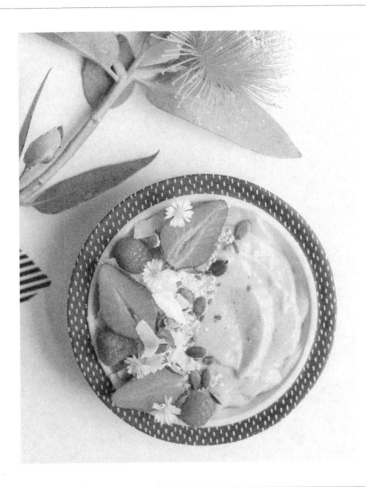

CARBS – 10 g   FAT – 0 g   PROTEIN – 1 g   CALORIES – 42

Ingredients

- *2 frozen bananas*
- *2 Tbsp dried organic goji berries*
- *1 medium apple, rinsed, cored and chopped*
- *½ cup cold water, to blend*
- *1 cup strawberries, rinsed*
- *¼ ripe avocado*
- *1 Tbsp fresh lemon juice*
- *1 tsp fresh root ginger, chopped*

Directions

1. Blend everything well.
2. Serve with preferred toppings.
3. Enjoy!

HERBAL TEA

SERVINGS: 20   PREP TIME: 5 min.   COOK TIME: 30 min.

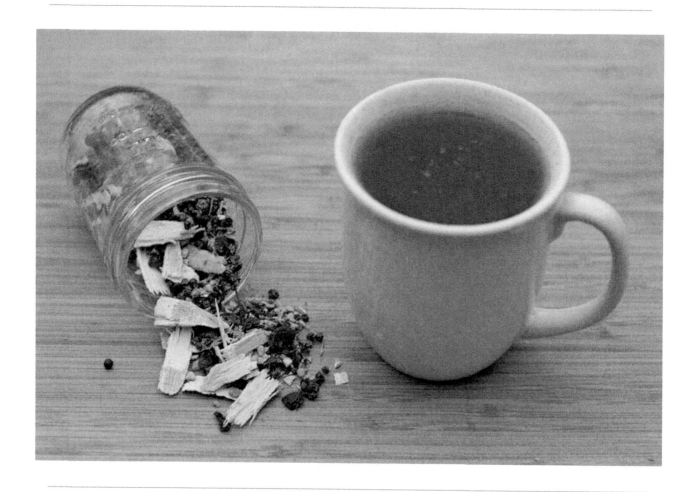

CARBS – 112 g   FAT – 8 g   PROTEIN – 5 g   CALORIES – 499

Ingredients

- *4 Tbsp dried elderberries*
- *4 Tbsp dried rose hips*
- *4 Tbsp echinacea root*
- *4 Tbsp astragalus*
- *4 Tbsp dried ginger*

Directions

1. Add all herbs to a mason jar.
2. Cover and shake well to combine.
3. 1-2 Tbsp of mixture will be enough for 1 cup of tea.
4. Add it to a small pot with water and simmer for 30 minutes. Strain the herbs.
5. Enjoy!

MANDARIN HERB TEA

SERVINGS: 2   PREP TIME: 5 min.   COOK TIME: 5 min.

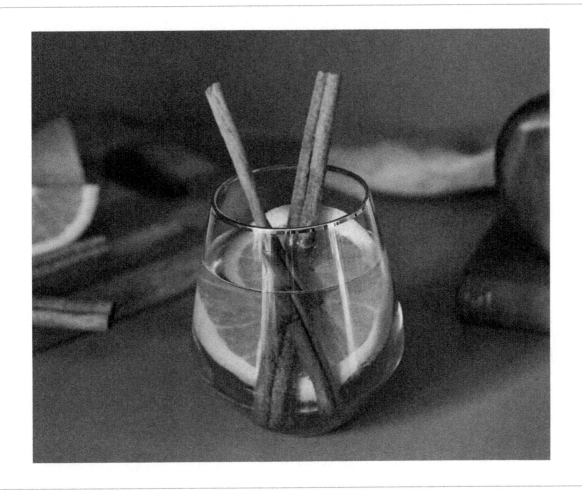

CARBS – 1 g   FAT – 0 g   PROTEIN – 1 g   CALORIES – 20

Ingredients

- *2 cups fresh water*
- *1 lemon, washed and sliced thick*
- *1 sunray mandarin orange, washed and sliced thick*
- *1 sprig fresh rosemary*
- *1 Tbsp honey*

Directions

1. Add water to a pot and let it boil.
2. Add lemon, orange , and rosemary.
3. Steep for 5 minutes, then strain.
4. Add honey and stir well.
5. Enjoy!

GOLDEN MILK CHAI

SERVINGS: 1   PREP TIME: 5 min.   COOK TIME: 5 min.

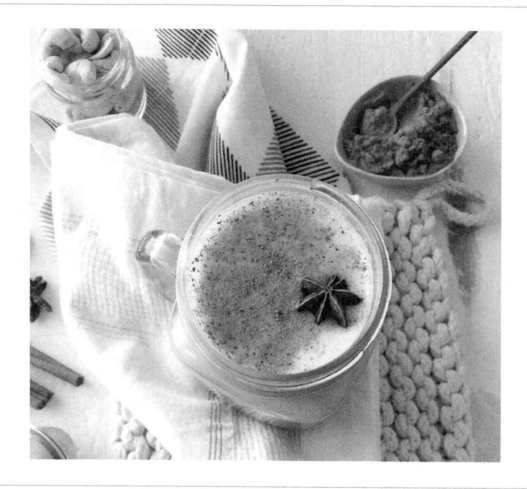

CARBS – 11 g   FAT – 2 g   PROTEIN – 3 g   CALORIES – 74

Ingredients

- *12 oz milk*
- *1 cinnamon stick*
- *2 star anise*
- *10 cardamom pods cracked opened*
- *10 whole cloves*
- *2 tsp ground turmeric*
- *½ tsp ground nutmeg plus more for topping*
- *10 black peppercorns*
- *1 tsp fennel seeds*
- *2 inches ginger, chopped*
- *1 tsp honey*
- *2 tsp loose leaf black tea*
- *1 tsp ghee*

Directions

1. Add 8 oz milk and all ingredients (except tea) to a small saucepan.
2. Heat on medium-low. Simmer for 10 minutes.
3. Turn off heat. Add loose-leaf tea.
4. Cover with lid and steep for 3 minutes.
5. Heat remaining milk and froth it.
6. Strain golden chai and top with frothed milk.
7. Sprinkle with nutmeg and cinnamon. Top with anise.
8. Enjoy!

BAOBAB CITRUS DRINK

SERVINGS: 1   PREP TIME: 5 min.   COOK TIME: 5 min.

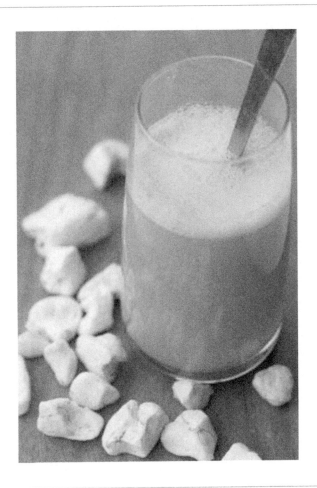

CARBS – 16 g   FAT – 0 g   PROTEIN – 1 g   CALORIES – 50

Ingredients

- *2-3 tsp Aduna Baobab Powder*
- *1 cup hot water*
- *1 wedge of lemon*
- *1 slice of ginger*

Directions

1. Mix baobab powder with 2 Tbsp cold water to get a smooth paste.
2. Boil the water and let cool for 1-2 minutes. Don't use boiling water because it will reduce the nutrition of the baobab.
3. Add hot water and stir well.
4. Squeeze lemon juice and add a slice of ginger.
5. Enjoy!

HOT CHOCOLATE

SERVINGS: 1   PREP TIME: 5 min.   COOK TIME: 3 min.

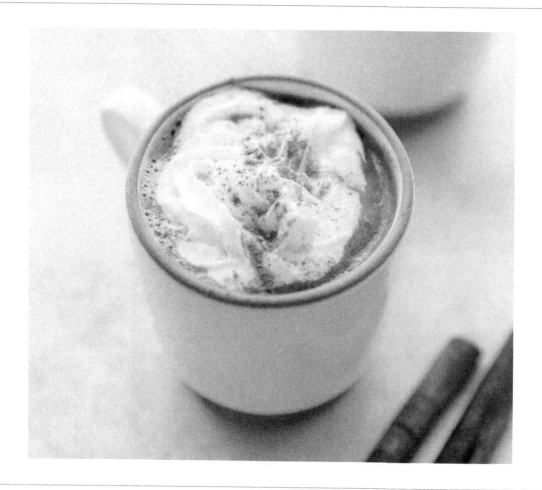

CARBS – 26 g   FAT – 5 g   PROTEIN – 8 g   CALORIES – 192

Ingredients

- *1 cup whole milk*
- *1 Tbsp raw cacao powder*
- *2 tsp honey*
- *½ tsp turmeric root, peeled and grated*
- *¼ tsp ground ginger*
- *¼ tsp ground cinnamon*
- *½ tsp coconut oil*

Directions

1. Add all ingredients to a small saucepan.
2. Heat over medium heat and simmer, occasionally stirring until spices and cocoa are mixed well and it's warmed through.
3. Enjoy!

GINGER LEMON TEA

SERVINGS: 1-2   PREP TIME: 5 min.   COOK TIME: 5 min.

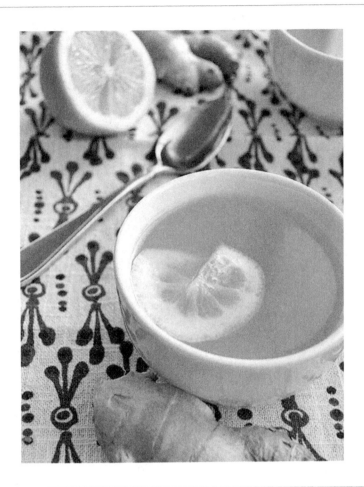

CARBS – 9 g   FAT – 0 g   PROTEIN – 0 g   CALORIES – 32

Ingredients

- *5 fresh sage leaves, ripped in half*
- *2 fresh thyme sprigs*
- *3 cm knob of ginger, sliced*
- *2 cups boiling water*
- *Juice of 1 lemon*
- *2 tsp sweetener of choice*

Directions

1. Put all ingredients (except sweetener) in a saucepan.
2. Let simmer for 4-5 minutes.
3. Strain the mixture and add sweetener.
4. Drink warm or cold.
5. Enjoy!

HOT TODDY

SERVINGS: 2   PREP TIME: 5 min.   COOK TIME: 5 min.

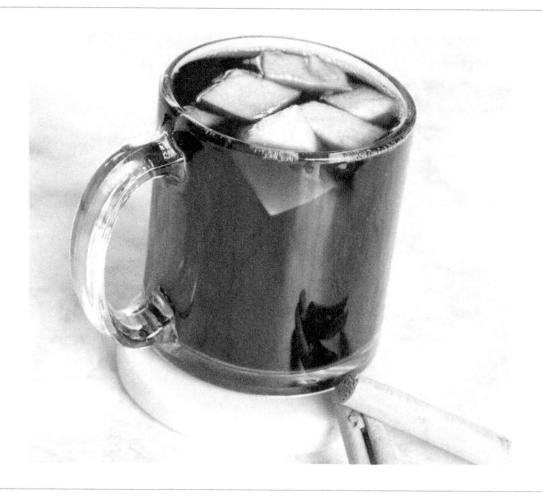

CARBS – 7 g   FAT – 0 g   PROTEIN – 0 g   CALORIES – 130

Ingredients

- *½ cup homemade cherry juice*
- *¼ cup organic raw apple cider vinegar*
- *1-inch ginger grated*
- *1 tsp honey*
- *1 tsp ground cinnamon*
- *1 dash ground clove*

Directions

1. Add cherry juice and ginger to a small saucepot. Bring to boil and simmer for 1-2 minutes.
2. Add apple cider vinegar and apples. Simmer for 2 minutes more.
3. Add clove, honey, and cinnamon. Simmer for 1 minute.
4. Enjoy!

TURMERIC TEA

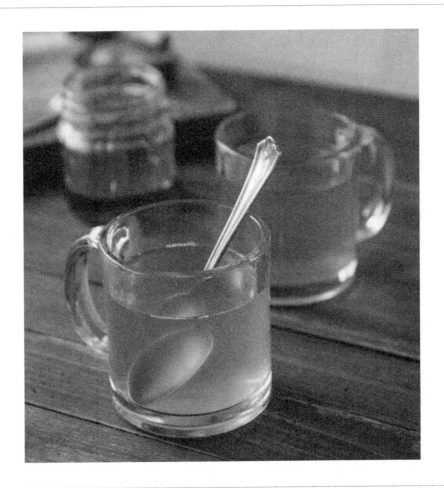

CARBS – 14 g   FAT – 0 g   PROTEIN – 0 g   CALORIES – 51

Ingredients

- *8 oz filtered water*
- *1-inch piece fresh ginger, sliced*
- *½ Tbsp honey*
- *¼ tsp turmeric powder*
- *½ medium lemon, juiced*
- *1 pinch cayenne pepper*

Directions

1. Combine ginger slices and hot water in a mug.
2. Steep for 3 minutes.
3. Add turmeric, honey, cayenne, and lemon juice.
4. Strain the tea with a sieve (optional).
5. Enjoy!

GINSENG TEA

SERVINGS: 2   PREP TIME: 5 min.   COOK TIME: 30 min.

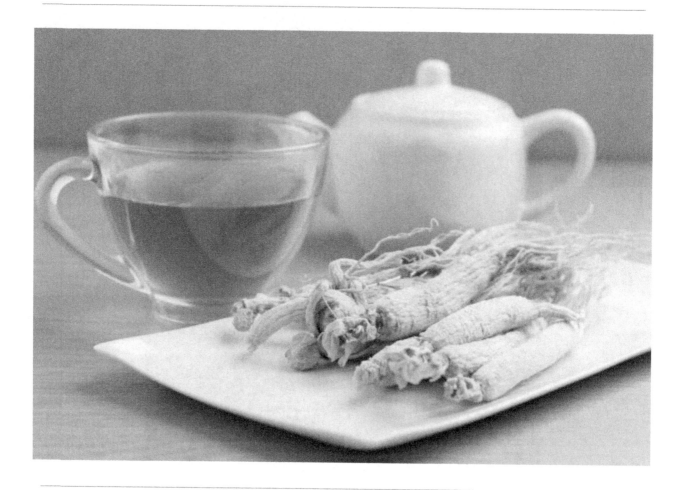

CARBS – 5 g   FAT – 0 g   PROTEIN – 0 g   CALORIES – 22

Ingredients

- *50 g fresh ginseng, rinsed properly*
- *1 dried jujube, rinsed*
- *500 ml water*
- *1 tsp honey*

Directions

1. Put the water into a pot. Add the ginseng and Chinese dates.
2. Let simmer on low heat for 20-25 minutes.
3. Serve!

ELDERBERRY TEA

SERVINGS: 2   PREP TIME: 5 min.   COOK TIME: 25 min.

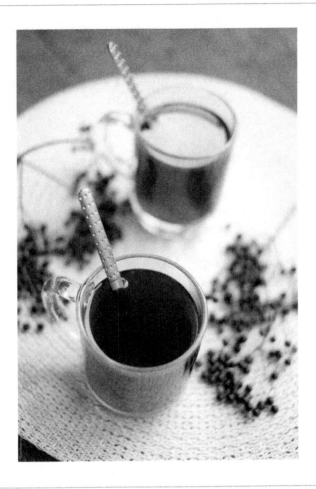

CARBS – 2 g   FAT – 0 g   PROTEIN – 0 g   CALORIES – 42

Ingredients

- 2 Tbsp dried elderberries
- 2 cups water
- 1 cinnamon stick
- 2 slices fresh ginger
- 1 tsp raw honey

Directions

1. Add all ingredients to a small saucepan.
2. Bring to a boil.
3. Simmer for 20 minutes on low heat.
4. Turn off and strain the tea.
5. Try to squeeze as much juice from elderberries as possible using a spoon.
6. When the tea has cooled some, add honey.
7. Enjoy!

CONCLUSION

Thank you for reading this book and having the patience to try the recipes.

I do hope that you have had as much enjoyment reading and experimenting with the meals as I have had writing the book.

If you would like to leave a comment, you can do so at the Order section->Digital orders, in your Amazon account.

Stay safe and healthy!

RECIPE INDEX

Dry Weights

OZ	(spoon)	C	(scale)	(scale)
1/2 OZ	1 Tbsp	1/16 C	15 g	
1 OZ	2 Tbsp	1/8 C	28 g	
2 OZ	4 Tbsp	1/4 C	57 g	
3 OZ	6 Tbsp	1/3 C	85 g	
4 OZ	8 Tbsp	1/2 C	115 g	1/4 lb
8 OZ	16 Tbsp	1 C	227 g	1/2 lb
12 OZ	24 Tbsp	1 1/2 C	340 g	3/4 lb
16 OZ	32 Tbsp	2 C	455 g	1 lb

Liquid Conversions

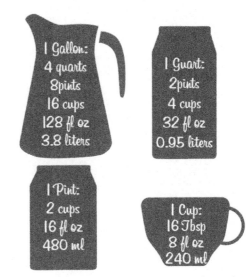

1 Gallon:
4 quarts
8 pints
16 cups
128 fl oz
3.8 liters

1 Quart:
2 pints
4 cups
32 fl oz
0.95 liters

1 Pint:
2 cups
16 fl oz
480 ml

1 Cup:
16 Tbsp
8 fl oz
240 ml

OZ	(spoon)	(spoon)	mL	C	Pt	Qt
1 oz	6 tsp	2 Tbsp	30 ml	1/8 C		
2 oz	12 tsp	4 Tbsp	60 ml	1/4 C		
2 2/3 oz	16 tsp	5 Tbsp	80 ml	1/3 C		
4 oz	24 tsp	8 Tbsp	120 ml	1/2 C		
5 1/3 oz	32 tsp	11 Tbsp	160 ml	2/3 C		
6 oz	36 tsp	12 Tbsp	177 ml	3/4 C		
8 oz	48 tsp	16 Tbsp	237 ml	1 C	1/2 pt	1/4 qt
16 oz	96 tsp	32 Tbsp	480 ml	2 C	1 pt	1/2 qt
32 oz	192 tsp	64 Tbsp	950 ml	4 C	2 pt	1 qt

Fahrenheit to Celcius (F to C)

500 F = 260 C
475 F = 245 C
450 F = 235 C
425 F = 220 C
400 F = 205 C
375 F = 190 C
350 F = 180 C
325 F = 160 C
300 F = 150 C
275 F = 135 C
250 F = 120 C
225 F = 107 C

1 tsp:
5 ml

1 Tbsp:
15 ml

Safe Cooking Meat Temperatures

Minimum temperatures:

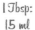

USDA Safe at 145 F   USDA Safe at 160 F   USDA Safe at 165 F

Beef Steaks, Briskets, and Roasts; Pork Chops, Roasts, Ribs, Shoulders, and Butts; Lamb Chops, Legs, and Roasts; Fresh Hams, Veal Steaks, Fish, and Shrimp

Ground Meats (except poultry)

Chicken & Turkey, ground or whole

Printed in Great Britain
by Amazon

37878667R00059